It's Not You
IT'S PERI MENOPAUSE

SARAH GRAY is one of Australia's leading dual-qualified health professionals in pharmacy and nutrition, and a certified menopause lifestyle practitioner with over 25 years of experience in the health and wellness industry. Her holistic approach focuses on supplements and science-based solutions for perimenopause and menopause. A trusted thought leader, Sarah has appeared on Channel 10's *My Market Kitchen* and is a recognised voice across radio, print, digital media and podcasts. She is also a regular contributor to leading health blogs and publications.

@the_nutrition_pharmacist

Praise for *It's Not You, It's Perimenopause*

'This book is a brilliant, science-backed guide to navigating perimenopause. As both a pharmacist and nutritionist, Sarah Gray brings a rare and valuable blend of expertise – grounding her advice in solid evidence while keeping it deeply practical. I especially love that she starts with nutrition and lifestyle foundations, then layers in supplement options where appropriate. With checklists, action plans, and clear explanations, *It's Not You, It's Perimenopause* is a reader-friendly, trustworthy resource – free from hype, fluff or fads. A must-read for any woman wanting real solutions during these years.'

—**Dr Joanna McMillan, Nutrition Scientist, TV Host, Speaker, Author and Food Futurist**

'Sarah Gray cuts through the confusion with clarity, compassion and clinical know-how. This is the guide I wish every woman had in her hands the moment (or even before) perimenopause begins. It's smart, accessible and genuinely empowering – grounded in science, but never overwhelming. With its structured, holistic approach and real-world case studies, *It's Not You, It's Perimenopause* doesn't just inform – it gives women a roadmap back to feeling like themselves again.'

—**Elizabeth Barbalich, BSc Biology, MBA, Qualified Naturopath, Founder & CEO of Antipodes® skincare**

'The heart of good healthcare is a desire to make a positive impact on a human being. That is Sarah Gray. Sarah is passionate about excellence in the science of health, founded by ethics and evidence. In this, she puts the person at the centre of her work. That is why this book is important. It's Not You, It's Perimenopause is an evidenced-based dive into navigating the transformative years for some of the most special people in the world – the women in our lives.'

—Dr. Dinesh Palipana OAM, doctor, lawyer, Queensland Australian of the Year, and author

'Sarah Gray has written the ultimate guide to navigating perimenopause with clarity, compassion, and confidence. Equal parts science and soul, this book demystifies what's happening to your body and gives you practical tools to feel like yourself again. Honest, relatable, and empowering, this is the must-have companion for every woman entering this transformative stage of life.'

—Kelly Irving, Book Coach, Editor and Founder of the Expert Author Community

'It's Not You, It's Perimenopause is an outstanding, science-based guide for women navigating midlife changes. Sarah blends clinical expertise with practical advice, offering clear, actionable steps without the confusion that often surrounds this life stage. I especially value her focus on gut health, an often overlooked but critical piece of the peri-puzzle, particularly for women seeking a lifestyle-first approach. With her engaging tone and evidence-based strategies, this book empowers women to take control of their health in a way that feels achievable and sustainable.'

—Nicole Dynan, Leading Gut Health Dietitian, Speaker & Media Commentator

'Sarah's dual expertise in both pharmacy and nutrition places her in a uniquely credible position, immediately earning the reader's trust. In It's Not You, It's Perimenopause, she offers an engaging, accessible, and empowering read. With a practical, easy-to-digest format, Sarah thoughtfully guides readers through the physical aspects of perimenopause – particularly the power of nourishment through food – while also addressing the often-overlooked emotional and mental shifts. From mindfulness to movement, her holistic approach offers a reassuring and relatable companion through this transformative life stage.'

—**Kelly Michelakis, Founder of The Hellenic Odyssey and an advocate of the Mediterranean diet**

'In It's Not You, It's Perimenopause, Sarah Gray delivers a goldmine of information, and practical strategies for women, and their loved ones, who are navigating perimenopause. Sarah's unique background in pharmacy and nutrition makes this book refreshingly clear, delivering information that is scientifically sound, and practical strategies that are genuinely helpful. I particularly enjoyed the use of case studies to help build connection; I am sure many of us can see some of ourselves in Sophia! This book is the perfect companion for women seeking real, effective support through this stage of life.'

—**Chloe McLeod, Founder & Speaker, Advanced Sports Dietitian and media spokesperson**

'If you are looking for science based answers to understanding perimenopause and menopause this book will definitely help you. Sarah shares stories to relate to and tips to help guide you through this tricky stage of life with a no fad, evidenced based approach.'

—**Simone Austin, Advanced Sports Dietitian, author, media spokesperson, speaker and public health advocate**

'It's Not You, It's *Perimenopause* is such a trustworthy and practical resource for anyone managing perimenopause. I love that it's based on solid science and evidence but written in a really approachable way that makes it easy to take action. The real standout for me is the case studies and the thread of Sophia's story throughout – they bring the lived experience to life and will help many readers feel less alone and truly seen. It's so refreshing to see the focus on lifestyle changes alongside supplements and medical support. It's such a well-rounded, balanced guide – a must-read!'

—Sonya Lovell, Speaker, Podcast Host and Advocate

It's Not You
IT'S PERI MENOPAUSE

SARAH GRAY

First published in 2025
Copyright © Sarah Gray 2025

All rights reserved. No part of this book may be reproduced or transmitted in any form or by any means, electronic or mechanical, including AI-generated reproductions, photocopying, recording, or by any information storage and retrieval system, without prior written permission from the publisher. The Australian *Copyright Act 1968* (the Act) allows a maximum of one chapter or 10 per cent of this book, whichever is the greater, to be photocopied by any educational institution for its educational purposes provided that the educational institution (or body that administers it) has given a remuneration notice to the Copyright Agency (Australia) under the Act.

A catalogue record for this book is available from the National Library of Australia

ISBN 978 1 7638009 8 4
eISBN 978 1 7638009 6 0

Cover design: Christa Moffitt, Christabella Designs
Author photo by Charlotte Jayasuriya, Location, Beauty Collective Co
Typeset in 10/17 pt Lora by Post Pre-press Group

The information contained in this book is provided for general guidance on the specific subjects addressed, but is not a substitute for, and should not be relied upon as, medical, healthcare, pharmaceutical, or other professional advice tailored to individual circumstances or locations. You should consult a registered GP for full medical clearance before making any changes discussed in this book. All health decisions remain the responsibility of the individual. The author and publisher claim no responsibility to any person or entity for any liability, loss or damage caused or alleged to be caused directly or indirectly as a result of the use, application or interpretation of the material in this book. Client case studies in this book are de-identified and fictionalised compilations of selected cases for the purposes of illustration only. Any resemblance to any real-life case is purely coincidental.

The Kind Press acknowledges all Aboriginal and Torres Strait Islander Traditional Custodians of Country and recognises their continuing connection to land, sea, culture and community. We pay our respects to Elders past and present.

For further information visit the author's website at
www.thenutritionpharmacist.com

For Hugo
You were my favourite hello and my hardest goodbye xx

CONTENTS

Introduction	1
What Makes This Book Different from Others	5
How to Use This Book	9
You Can Feel Like Yourself Again	11

PART I: UNDERSTANDING THE FUNDAMENTALS

Chapter 1: What Is Perimenopause?	15
Clinical case: Raquel's revelation	37
Chapter 2: Assess Yourself and Set Clear Goals	39
Clinical case: Danielle's discovery	56

PART II: SCIENCE-BASED SOLUTIONS

Chapter 3: Nutrition Tools and Tactics	61
Tactic 1: Level up your protein	64
Tactic 2: Choose smart carbs	69
Tactic 3: Crowd your plate with plant foods	71
Tactic 4: Balance your hormones with phytoestrogens	74
Tactic 5: Omega-3s for brain and heart health	78
Tactic 6: Eat energy-boosting foods	79
Tactic 7: Stay well hydrated, and limit caffeine and alcohol	81
Tactic 8: Nourish your gut health	83
Tactic 9: Calcium plus D for strong bones	86
Clinical case: Emma's evolution	103

Chapter 4: Lifestyle Shifts That Make a Difference — 105
Tactic 1: Self-care, meditation and mindfulness — 108
Tactic 2: Establish a sleep routine — 110
Tactic 3: Regular exercise — 112
Tactic 4: Limit endocrine-disrupting chemicals — 115
Tactic 5: Medical treatments — 118
Clinical case: Melanie's momentum — 131

Chapter 5: Smart Supplement Strategies — 133
Step 1: Know your bloodwork — 135
Step 2: Alleviate specific symptoms — 136
Step 3: Support your body in this transition — 136
General supportive supplements — 140
Hormonal-symptom support supplements — 150
Energy support supplements — 155
Stress, sleep and mood-support supplements — 158
Clinical case: Olivia's overwhelm — 164

PART III: FROM PLAN TO ACTION

Chapter 6: Create Your Perimenopause Action Plan — 167

Bonus Chapter: How to Build a Peri-Healthy Plate — 181
How to build a peri-healthy meal — 182
Peri-healthy breakfast recipes — 184
Peri-healthy lunch recipes — 186
Peri-healthy dinner recipes — 188
Peri-healthy snack guide — 191

Recipe notes — 194
Beyond this book — 195
Acknowledgments and gratitude — 199
References — 201
About the author — 215

INTRODUCTION

Welcome to *It's Not You, It's Perimenopause*, your trusted guide when it comes to dealing with troublesome midlife symptoms caused by hormonal changes. I wrote this book to help women like you navigate all the shifts that come with perimenopause. You no longer have to suffer in silence and overwhelm.

• • • • • • • • • • • • •

SOPHIA hears the alarm clock and lifts her heavy head off the pillow to face yet another grinding day in the Lowe household. Here goes. Time to get Zoe ready for school, feed the dogs, serve breakfast, wave hubby goodbye and maybe fit in a quick thirty-minute cardio workout – otherwise imagine what her midline would look like. After three deep breaths, she rises to an argument from headstrong Zoe and barking pups desperately wanting their morning freedom. No wonder she is exhausted before the day has begun.

In the words of Dr Jason, 'you are tired all the time because you are too busy'. HR can be such a draining job, and this is probably the icing on the cake in a hectic lifestyle that feels devoid of any self-care or enjoyment. What is it they say? *Life starts at 40. Yeah, right.*

After rushing around all morning, Sophia takes a moment to guzzle down a superfood smoothie her Pilates instructor swears by. *It tastes gross!* But if this is the price to pay to get her body of ten years ago back, she will do it. Her smoothie is the perfect fluid vehicle to help slip down the array of colourful vitamin pills, as well as a liquid herbal tonic that is supposed to help control her sugar cravings. Didn't seem to help last night as she devoured half a block of chocolate. *Felt like a good idea at the time.*

Time to walk to the station and head to the office. *Must get those 10,000 steps up.* On the train, Sophia has some 'me time' and thinks about how she is feeling. Her eyes close as she feels a wave of fatigue so intense she could lie down between the seats and have a nap. This happens at least three times a day, but no need to worry, Dr Jase seems to think it's 'normal at your age'. And what about those wild mood fluctuations? One minute she feels calm and in control, next minute she is in a flood of tears and rage, like when Chris moved her phone charger last night. *But that is super annoying.*

She thinks about her waistline as her once-loose work trousers dig in against her soft flesh, actually causing a bit of pain. But there is NO way she will be buying a size up. She is already two sizes up from last year. Maybe this cardio routine, superfood regime and endless vitamins are not really helping? Sophia takes a deep breath, closes her eyes and thinks, *I'll do whatever it takes to feel like my old self again, no matter the cost.* She looks up and notices she missed her station for the office. *Great, another day in the glorious life of Sophia. Let's go.*

• • • • • • • • • • • •

Meet Sophia. I write more about her throughout this book. She's a fictional character representing the collection of women I have helped over the years. Did some of her story resonate with you? At your wits' end with perimenopause symptoms with no viable solutions in sight? All too often, I hear stories like Sophia's and I'm sure this is the same for you.

INTRODUCTION

It's time to take control back of our health so we can prosper, even when it feels like nothing really makes a difference.

Even when we think, *maybe this is all in my head?* I can assure you it's not. For us women, middle age comes with a unique group of challenges. All of a sudden, our bodies feel different, and we begin to wonder if this is the way it will be from now on.

Have you noticed more belly fat, despite not really changing your diet or exercise?

Have you noticed less tone in your muscles, even though you are exercising more?

Have you noticed wild fluctuations in mood, or more frequent bouts of sweating, brain fog and fatigue?

Perhaps your period is arriving unexpectedly after not coming for months, or you're back to the same level of period paid as when you were at school?

No doubt some, or maybe all these things, sound familiar. If so, you can rest assured that other women of a similar age are also experiencing these shifts. It's a new phase of life, perimenopause. Part of the privilege of ageing is to witness changes like this in your body over time.

Let's be honest, there's no sugarcoating it, this is hard. It's hard to feel like someone else in your own skin. It's hard to feel out of control when it comes to feelings of rage, anger and sadness – all in a few minutes. It's even harder when no one can explain why you feel this way, especially when you read about it and it feels like you have to be a scientist to understand it all. You may have even considered hiring an assistant to keep track of all the suggested diet changes, supplements, exercise and more. All the while, it's difficult to feel alone, isolated and lost when it comes to what to do next, who to ask, and more importantly, who you can trust when it comes to advice. While many symptoms and emotions are likely inevitable, you do not have to suffer alone or in silence.

There are science-based solutions that can help you feel like you again. There's also light ahead. Perimenopause is a life phase – it's not forever – lasting on average around four to eight years.

Like Sophia, have you questioned why this is all happening and seemingly all at once? In a snapshot, most symptoms can be linked to changes in hormone levels as you age. It all starts with a drop in the key hormone progesterone (your body makes less), together with wildly fluctuating oestrogen. This triggers a range of symptoms that leave you feeling, well, let's say, far from the best version of you.

It may be comforting to realise you are not alone. A community, albeit a silent one, of women around you is feeling the same. Medical publications state that perimenopause starts in your 40s. But in reality, women can experience symptoms from their mid-30s. It's estimated that almost 7 million women in Australia are peri-menopausal or menopausal. Around 2 million of those women report moderate to severe symptoms that impact their quality of life. So, next time you're out for a ladies' lunch, don't be afraid to open up. Together you can support each other. Research backs this up. A strong sense of community and connectedness is beneficial for mental and physical wellbeing.

WHAT MAKES THIS BOOK DIFFERENT FROM OTHERS

Five years ago, hardly anyone had even heard the word perimenopause. Now it is part of everyday vernacular, and that, my friends, is a great thing. More awareness leads to more support, resources, conversations and progression. But it can also lead to misinformation, overwhelm and confusion, as you are served up too many solutions that seem complex, expensive and sometimes contradictory. Should you try intermittent fasting? Or did you just read that it might not be good for middle-aged women after all? What about magnesium? Does it cure every single symptom of perimenopause? Or is it all just hype? And then there's the ongoing debate about Hormone Replacement Therapy (HRT). Is it safe or not?

After spending over twenty-five years in the health and wellness industry, I have seen it all. Confusion often leads people to dismiss everything. Most information is too scientific for us to understand and know what to do next. Many of the women who come to me for help have already given up, feel defeated, accept they need to push through this phase or are hoping it just goes away. So, despite there being an abundance of books, articles, social media pages, podcasts and more, many women are suffering on a daily basis.

This book is different.

You don't need a science degree to understand it, a bank loan to fund the remedies, or an extra day in the week to implement all the tactics. The information is easy to digest and always science-based. It will:

1. Help you identify and understand your most troublesome symptoms such as midline weight gain, brain fog, mood swings, changes to your period, hot flushes and night sweats, trouble sleeping, vaginal dryness, decreased libido and joint pain.

2. Leave you with a personalised perimenopause Action Plan that is easy to implement and actually works.

My hope is that by the end of this book, you will feel like you are entering a new phase of life. With my vast experience as a uniquely qualified pharmacist and nutritionist, I personally guide you through perimenopause. I have spent over two decades helping women understand more about their health, and I arm you with the confidence you need to navigate your health journey like a boss! Using my experience and learnings, I have developed a unique approach that actually has a noticeable impact on your life and wellbeing. The tactics in this book draw upon all areas of my experience and knowledge, and everything shared is evidence-based. No fad diets or fast fixes. Strap yourself in for a fun-filled, realistic ride that helps you better manage perimenopause symptoms, whatever they may be in your case.

Through small and impactful changes to diet and lifestyle and with the role of supplements to support in reaching your goals, I leave you with true insight about the way supplements work, the evidence, and how you can maximise your choices to reap the benefits. No more wasting money on an expensive pee! I also

WHAT MAKES THIS BOOK DIFFERENT FROM OTHERS

guide you on the many benefits of HRT, and how you can open a conversation with your doctor, if appropriate for you.

So, if you've ever found yourself staring at the mega aisle of supplements at the supermarket, if you've ever been lured in by an influencer who eliminated hot flushes with a herbal tonic, or if you've simply thrown caution to the wind and purchased that magnesium supplement in the hope your belly fat will disappear in days, or debated with your friends about the safety of HRT, well, this is the book for you. Now before I go on, I have to say, it's not all doom and gloom. The positive? There are many nutritional tactics, supplements, treatments and lifestyle approaches that have evidence to show they help alleviate perimenopause symptoms. Let's hero those that have evidence, and tread with caution where the evidence is lacking or yet to emerge. Let's completely avoid anything with zero evidence, despite what the fancy packaging and Instagram page are selling you.

News flash! This is not a weight-loss book. *It's Not You, It's Perimenopause* is designed to help you conquer troublesome perimenopause symptoms. If weight loss is a goal, then that's for you, but if you want sound sleep, better energy levels or less brain fog, then you will work towards that. So, get yourself a cuppa, sit back, and enjoy the ride. It's time to take back your power and thrive in perimenopause.

> **While you have probably tried what seems like every path that exists to see change with no success, I want to assure you there are evidence-based tactics you can implement every day to see noticeable results.**

HOW TO USE THIS BOOK

In Chapter 1, you learn about what is happening to your body during perimenopause. This provides a nice baseline to help understand why you are experiencing symptoms, respecting that your body is handling a lot for you as change happens.

In Chapter 2, you complete a self-assessment quiz to determine what is causing you the most distress, then gauge what stage you're at on the perimenopause journey.

Chapters 3, 4 and 5 showcase my recommended tactics when it comes to nutrition, lifestyle and supplements, guiding you on the science-backed tactics to weave into your daily life to alleviate symptoms and feel like yourself again.

In Chapter 6, you create your very own perimenopause Action Plan, using science-backed solutions to manage those symptoms.

When you see an Action Step, it is a cue to pause, a key step to take, even if you have time to do nothing else. This helps propel you forward and increases the chances of success.

Throughout the pages, you'll read client stories that are fictionalised, based on my real cases with identifying names and some details changed to protect privacy.

YOU CAN FEEL LIKE YOURSELF AGAIN

It's time to manage the symptoms of perimenopause by walking through the processes so you can thrive. With your dedication to prioritising your health and making changes in a consistent and kind way, you will feel better. Change does take time and by applying these small and clever tactics, your body will start to flourish.

> Close your eyes for a moment.
> Imagine that you feel light, energetic, happy and confident.
> Your daily brain fog has subsided.
> You have the energy to exercise, socialise and enjoy life.
> What once seemed impossible is now achievable.
> You see changes in your body and mind that you've yearned for.
>
> The noisy clutter of food groups to eliminate, and supplements and health trends to jump on, all fades into the distance.

It's time to create your unique Action Plan, where you feel like you again.

Part 1
UNDERSTANDING THE FUNDAMENTALS

Perimenopause is a time when everything changes and often without warning, when life is already filled with commitments, family, work and day-to-day tasks. It's also an important time to acknowledge that the body is undergoing change within.

Perimenopause is a major life transition. To appreciate that statement some more, it's good to get a handle on the main aspects, while not needing to be an absolute expert. This helps with acceptance and allows us to show kindness to the changes in this major life transitional phase. This is why we begin Part I by focusing on the fundamentals. Knowledge brings power. Once you understand the fundamentals, you can see why you need to change the operating rhythm across nutrition and lifestyle to support your body through to the other side. It's also key for getting a handle on the common threads of symptoms that are causing the most life disturbance. We do that with a quick self-assessment quiz. In this part, you plan and build upon a personal Action Plan. You not only assess where you're at now, but you set clear goals to work towards which will also be a measure for how you're feeling on the other side of the process where you can thrive in midlife and beyond.

Chapter 1

WHAT IS PERIMENOPAUSE?

• • • • • • • • • • • • •

Time to get ready for Chris' big 4-0 party.

Sophia sets up at the dining table and gets to work on a photo board. Old school, she knows, but everyone likes a good old-fashioned photo. She picks up a photo from their holiday to Bali around five years ago. Sophia can barely recognise herself. She was so much thinner and brighter. It's night and day from how she looks and feels right now. Will she ever feel like herself again? It seems this 'peri' era has well and truly commenced, and she will probably never feel like that bright, bubbly woman enjoying the poolside cocktail in Ubud.

This week has been a nightmare, starting with her period being so heavy she could barely function and the cramps reminding her of the ones she used to have at school. It left her feeling tired and more grumpy than usual. Then there's the 3 am wake-ups every single night. *What's that all about? It has to be caused by hormonal imbalances, right?* It's all her girlfriends talk about these days. But what does it really mean? *Isn't menopause when you lose all your female hormones or something?* Most of the information online goes right over Sophia's head.

And you can forget about knowing where to start when it comes to feeling better. Sophia knows she is a fad-diet, fast-fix kinda girl which probably hasn't helped her cause. She has tried so many so-called 'solutions' for her symptoms, and to be frank, nothing has made a noticeable difference.

• • • • • • • • • • • • •

Sophia's journey is one I hear almost daily in my work with women. In a world of information overload, you can often be left feeling confused and in overwhelm. A common question women ask me is, 'Where do I even start?' I truly believe it's important to arm yourself with a baseline of knowledge when it comes to health. But you don't need to be a scientist (unless you really want to, of course). To start this journey together, let's explore the fundamentals of what is happening in your body at this phase of life.

Firstly, it can be a comfort to appreciate your body for all the work it does for you. The symptoms you are experiencing are a normal physiological process. In essence, it's your body's way of coping with some serious hormonal changes and more. It can help to break down some of these major changes, how they impact different systems in your body, and why they cause a variety of effects such as weight gain, energy loss, mood swings, elevated stress and sleep disturbances, to name a few. In fact, there is a very long list of different symptoms of perimenopause, affecting almost all bodily systems. Understanding some of the key areas of change can help you better appreciate what's going on, especially on the inside.

So, what is perimenopause?

Put simply, perimenopause is a series of events that is a normal life phase for a woman. It usually spans four to eight years, but each

WHAT IS PERIMENOPAUSE?

individual has a unique experience and the duration and severity of symptoms is extremely variable. Perimenopause can arrive as early as your mid-30s or as late as your early-50s. It is a very personal journey. Before we dive in, it's interesting to note that not all women experience symptoms of perimenopause and the degree of symptoms varies for those who do. It is estimated that 20 percent have no symptoms, 60 percent experience mild to moderate symptoms and 20 percent have severe symptoms that impact daily life.

To understand what is happening in your body, it can help to briefly reflect back to earlier life, where you have likely experienced a natural menstrual cycle. Now keep in mind this is a general explanation to set the scene, not taking into account many individual variabilities. What you want to digest is what's happening to hormone levels, so you can see the stark differences as you enter perimenopause.

Your typical 28-day cycle is moderated by hormones, starting with day 1 marked as the first day you get your period. Between days 1 and 14, the pituitary gland in your brain releases Follicle-Stimulating Hormone (FSH) signalling the ovaries to prepare an egg for ovulation. This triggers an increase in the hormone oestrogen, which peaks just before ovulation, around day 14. Around day 14 (or mid-cycle) the pituitary releases a surge of Luteinizing Hormone (LH) which triggers the release of an egg. Ovulation is a term that describes the release of an egg from your ovary so it can travel to the uterus. After ovulation, between days 14 and 28, if pregnancy has not occurred, the levels of hormone progesterone rise and then fall again. At the same time, oestrogen levels trend downwards. Around day 28, levels of oestrogen and progesterone drop, and menstruation starts again.

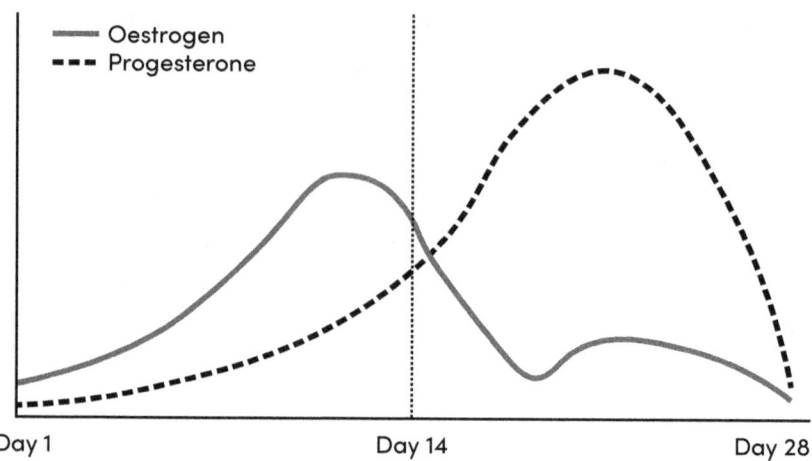

Note – *image is not to scale and simply represents the hormone trends*

In the perimenopause phase, and yes, it is just a phase (which can be helpful to remember; it won't last forever), your ovaries are winding down and beginning to run out of viable eggs. We are born with a finite number of eggs that steadily decreases over time. This means that each month when your pituitary gland releases FSH and LH, the ovaries do not always respond, as they are struggling to produce and release eggs. This leads to key hormonal changes. You will make less progesterone and start to release different levels of oestrogen than you used to. The balance of oestrogen becomes erratic, with wild fluctuations occurring on a daily basis.

These changes result in a raft of symptoms, the main one being erratic or irregular periods. Other symptoms can include vaginal dryness, changes in mood, irritability, anxiety, weight gain, hot flushes, night sweats and problems sleeping. Most people associate these kinds of symptoms with menopause itself. But you may be surprised to learn that the most varying and troublesome symptoms usually occur in perimenopause.

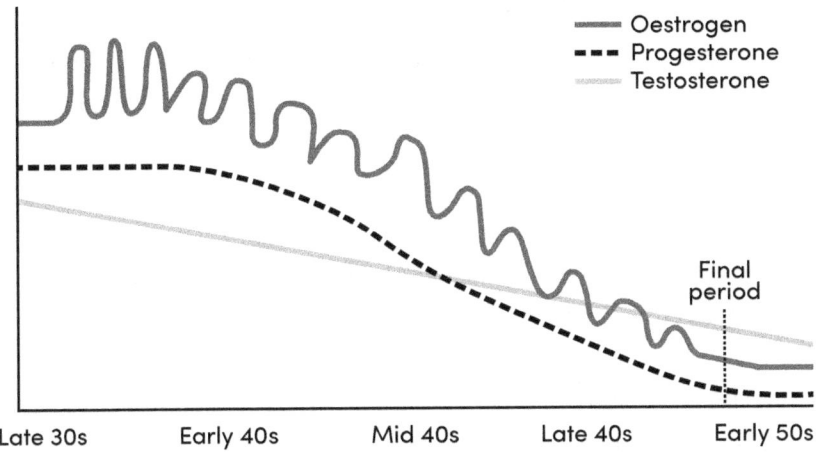

Note – *image is not to scale and simply represents the hormone trends*

There are a few things to be aware of as not all women will take this course in their lifespan. There are some cases of earlier onset symptoms, which can be the result of different factors.

Premature ovarian insufficiency

Around 4 percent of women will experience what is called premature or primary ovarian insufficiency (POI). This is when the ovaries stop working as they should before the age of 40. The ovaries do not release eggs or make the usual amounts of oestrogen. This can cause irregular or missed periods for many years.

Premature menopause

This is when menopause is reached before the age of 40. While this may be due to POI, it can also be a result of cancer treatments or surgical menopause, like removal of the ovaries or hysterectomy, which may be due to cancer or other health conditions like severe endometriosis.

The perimenopause stages

To break it down even further, there are a few stages of the perimenopause transition, but remember, these vary and are not the same for each person.

Very early perimenopause
Periods may still come like clockwork, or you may notice they are slightly irregular. Common symptoms at this stage:

- Heavy periods
- Increased period pain
- Sleep disturbances
- Mood changes
- Migraines

Early perimenopause
Periods or cycles start to become a lot more irregular. Common symptoms at this stage:

- Hot flushes
- Night sweats
- Heavy periods
- Mood changes
- Irritability
- Weight gain

Late perimenopause
Cycles become longer, and periods come further and further apart. Common symptoms at this stage:

- Worsening hot flushes
- Night sweats
- Aches and pains
- Vaginal dryness
- Brain fog
- Fatigue
- Low libido
- Weight gain

WHAT IS PERIMENOPAUSE?

What do your hormones do for you?

Here are some of the main roles that the three key hormones – oestrogen, progesterone and testosterone – play in your health. While this is not an exhaustive summary, it demonstrates how important these hormones are.

Oestrogen

Prior to menopause, the body produces a type of oestrogen called oestradiol. As oestrogen receptors are found throughout the body, including the reproductive tract, breasts, bone, brain, liver, colon, skin, salivary glands and more, the effects are wide reaching. Oestrogen plays a role in regulating your menstrual cycles, supporting a healthy metabolism, reducing inflammation, building muscle and bone, and helping to maintain things like your skin's moisture, mood, brain and heart health.

Progesterone

Your body relies on progesterone for many different processes and functions, such as helping regulate menstrual cycles, supporting a healthy metabolism, having a calming effect on the brain, reducing inflammation, supporting immune health, preventing bone loss, modulating libido and protecting the heart.

Testosterone

Levels of testosterone decline as you age and trend downwards as perimenopause progresses. Often, women experience more pronounced symptoms of low testosterone towards the later stages of perimenopause. These include low libido, thinning hair, muscle weakness, mood swings, fatigue, weight gain, and poor memory and concentration. Testosterone plays a role in regulating libido, bone and muscle health, heart health, mood, energy and sleep.

What is menopause?

Menopause is defined as the point in time when you have gone twelve consecutive months without a period. By the time you arrive here, your ovaries are producing very little oestrogen or progesterone and no longer have eggs to release, so you are unable to fall pregnant. At this stage, the rollercoaster settles somewhat, and you are almost ready to get off the ride! As your hormones start to stabilise, you may notice fewer symptoms until they completely disappear for some. Again, this is variable, and some women may continue to experience symptoms in the postmenopausal phase for a longer duration than others.

Perimenopause symptoms unpacked

Many different symptoms can appear as you move through the stages of perimenopause. When women come to me for help, their top concerns are weight gain, heavy periods, reduced energy levels, brain fog, sleep disturbances, mood changes, aches and pains, and higher levels of stress and anxiety. However, all experience a range of symptoms, caused by high or low levels of hormones, which change rapidly as their bodies adjust. While we will only deep-dive into some of the most common symptoms in this chapter, the following table summarises more areas of change you might experience. Perimenopause looks different for every woman and doesn't fit nicely into one box.

WHAT IS PERIMENOPAUSE?

LOW OESTROGEN

Less frequent periods	Brain fog	Dry skin
Lighter periods	Poor concentration	Midline weight gain
Night sweats	Low mood	Joint pain
Trouble sleeping	Mood swings	Fatigue
Vaginal dryness	Anxiety	Low libido

HIGH OESTROGEN

Low mood	Breast tenderness	Weight gain
Irritability	Bloating	Fatigue

LOW PROGESTERONE

Premenstrual syndrome	Spotting between cycles	Low libido
Irregular or missed periods	Heavy periods	Mood swings and irritability
Breast pain and tenderness	Fluid retention	Hot flushes
	Trouble sleeping	Fluid retention
	Anxiety	

HIGH PROGESTERONE

Low mood	Irritability	Dizziness

LOW TESTOSTERONE

Low libido	Hair thinning	Poor memory and concentration
Muscle weakness	Fatigue	
Mood swings and irritability	Weight gain	

* Common symptoms experienced by women. This table is not exhaustive, and other symptoms may be apparent from person to person.

Inflammation and perimenopause

One of the driving forces behind many symptoms of perimenopause is inflammation. The gradual decline in oestrogen and other factors leaves the body in a state of chronic, low-grade inflammation, which has been associated with many of the symptoms and changes occurring in your body. Many of the tactics we explore in Chapters 3, 4 and 5 help reduce levels of inflammation through diet, lifestyle and supplements.

Why is weight gain so common?

This is the million-dollar question, right? Why does it seem that as you get older, you are gaining weight while not necessarily eating more? And this despite hitting the gym or working out the same amount as when you were younger, or maybe even more? Your metabolism is not quite the same as it was in your 20s, meaning you start to experience changes in body shape and composition. Let's break this all down so you can better understand the 'why'.

Hormonal and physiological changes and weight

The tendency to easily gain weight, especially around the midline, is linked to key hormonal changes, as well as genetic and lifestyle changes that occur as women age. While hormonal factors contribute to changes in body composition in midlife, other factors are also at play. Firstly, it is a natural progression to lose muscle mass with age, while the proportion of fat in your body increases. As you lose muscle, this slows down your metabolism, which dictates the amount of energy your body burns at any given time, potentially causing weight gain even while your dietary and lifestyle patterns remain largely unchanged. This can feel frustrating, but rest assured there are things you can do about it.

Prior to menopause, women are naturally predisposed to

storing fat around the hips and thighs. Once oestrogen levels drop, this triggers a change in your body, and fat is now stored more around the waist and belly area, known as visceral fat. Visceral fat is linked with specific health impacts such as an increased risk of heart disease, type 2 diabetes, breast cancer and dementia. At the same time, all these changes to weight can be more or less significant for you, depending somewhat on genetics. For example, did your mother or grandmother experience stubborn belly fat as they entered this phase of life?

Oestrogen dominance and weight gain

Hormonal changes in perimenopause are key when it comes to unexpected weight gain. Progesterone levels usually decline first and do so at a faster rate than the gradual decline in oestrogen. This means you can often experience relative oestrogen dominance in this life stage. This may surprise you, as many think perimenopause is all about losing oestrogen.

Oestrogen dominance contributes to excess weight gain, a very common symptom of perimenopause. At the same time, the distribution of fat to the abdominal area is influenced by the overall decline of oestrogen. The liver plays a role here as well. It helps your body break down oestrogen which is beneficial when it's present in excess. However, if you are overweight or obese, this can increase the risk of liver disease or dysfunction making it harder for your body to eliminate oestrogen effectively.

As you can see, it is a complex interplay.

Gut health and weight

Key changes in gut health might impact weight during this era. Research suggests that your gut microbiome alters during menopause. Essentially, the gut microbiome is the collection of all the microbes in your gut which influences your body's response to foods and is important for your overall health. When this changes composition, it may impact the way your body metabolises food, making you more prone to weight gain.

Metabolic changes and weight

Then there's the impact of hormonal changes on the way your body metabolises fat and sugar. Evidence shows that the ageing process, together with hormonal changes, may cause insulin resistance. Insulin resistance affects your body's ability to use insulin efficiently. Put simply, insulin is a hormone that reduces the level of glucose, a type of sugar, in your blood. If you have insulin resistance, you may have higher levels of sugar in your blood which could lead to weight gain.

Sleep and weight

You may also be surprised that changes in sleep patterns around perimenopause may cause weight gain. It is thought that sleep disturbances may impact the way your body metabolises fat, which could increase fat storage, leading to weight gain.

So, as you can see, there is no one single reason why you may find yourself with excess midline fat that you cannot seem to shift. Your body is managing a lot of change. As we progress, you will learn how to support yourself and your body so that the impact on your waist is minimal.

Why can periods be heavier?

While it can be hard to define heavy periods from woman to woman, there are common signs. Do you have to change your tampon or pad every hour or so, or empty your menstrual cup more regularly? Are you doubling up on sanitary products like using a tampon and a pad? These are sure-fire signs that your menstrual blood loss is increasing. During perimenopause, heavy bleeding is not unusual as levels of oestrogen and progesterone change. It is important to remember that these are the primary hormones that regulate your menstrual cycle. One of the main concerns with increased blood loss is the potential for iron deficiency, which we will address in later chapters.

The impact on energy levels, sleep and stress

Do you ever feel like a nanna nap in the middle of the day? Anxious? Waking multiple times in a hot sweat? Many women in midlife experience some or all of these symptoms. Why is this so? As you might now expect, some key hormonal changes can explain most of these symptoms. Not surprisingly, a 2022 online survey of women over 40 found that nearly 67 percent experienced regular fatigue and 62 percent reported feeling anxious. So, what exactly is causing this? As is often the case with perimenopause, there is not one simple answer. Instead, there is an interplay of systems and processes, each contributing in different ways to the fatigue and, in some cases, sheer exhaustion that many women report.

Reflect on what is happening within your body. Progesterone levels are declining, oestrogen is wildly fluctuating, and testosterone is gradually decreasing over time. These hormonal changes can disrupt your daily rhythm, often leaving you feeling tired, drained and quite frankly, completely worn out. This imbalance has a noticeable impact on sleep quality. Hot flushes and night sweats may become more frequent, disturbing your ability to rest and sleep. Changing hormone levels affect the brain's ability to regulate body temperature. It's as though your internal thermostat is faulty, triggering sudden bouts of heat, or a flushed face, and excessive sweating as your body attempts to cool down.

Then there are changes to the main stress hormone called

cortisol. Oestrogen helps to buffer the levels of cortisol, preventing it from getting too high. With fluctuations of oestrogen, this means cortisol cannot be regulated as well as it used to be. As time goes by, your levels of cortisol naturally increase which leaves you more stressed, anxious, irritable and feeling constantly on edge. It also plays with your body clock, further reducing sleep quality and leaving you feeling less than your best come morning time.

It's also worth mentioning changes in levels of melatonin, which can particularly impact sleep quality. Melatonin is the hormone that helps regulate your sleep patterns. Levels normally rise at night when it is dark and fall during the morning when it becomes light. As you age, levels of melatonin naturally drop, impacting your ability to get good quality shut-eye.

> **MELATONIN is a hormone that helps synchronise your internal sleep-wake clock – it lets the body know it's time for rest.**

Why do you experience mood swings?

Mood changes can cause daily disruptions in this phase of life. In fact, some women describe their changing moods as similar to, or even worse than, premenstrual syndrome. There can be periods of rage or extreme irritability, followed by low energy, tearfulness and low mood.

✱ If you are feeling low, and your mood changes are impacting your day-to-day life, you should speak to your doctor as soon as possible.

With wildly fluctuating oestrogen and declining levels of the more calming progesterone, it's no wonder you sometimes feel the extremes when it comes to mood. However, other things are also happening here. Hormonal changes have an impact on the serotonin levels in your brain. Serotonin, the happy hormone, is a chemical messenger in the brain that promotes feelings of happiness and wellbeing. While the research is still building in this space, it is believed that changes to oestrogen levels may lead to lower levels of serotonin. This might be responsible for feelings of distress, anger, panic, low energy levels and insomnia.

> **SEROTONIN,** known as the happy hormone, is the brain's messenger to promote happiness and wellbeing.

Can you blame hormone changes for brain fog?

Have you found yourself forgetting why you walked into a room, or always misplacing your keys or phone? Maybe lost for words mid-sentence? This is what brain fog can feel like. And yes, it is likely that fluctuating hormones are to blame, but the exact reason why it occurs is yet to be well-nailed down. We know oestrogen plays a key role in brain health. As the levels decline, the brain cells don't fire as well as they used to. The good news here is that this symptom is temporary for most women, and usually settles as their hormones do.

Why the new aches and pains?

Aching muscles and joints are another common symptom of perimenopause. One explanation is related to the anti-inflammatory effects of oestrogen and progesterone. As levels fall, you may experience new joint, muscle and tendon pain.

Other changes to be aware of

This is probably a good time to mention that oestrogen plays protective roles in earlier years, and when levels decline, this can increase your risk of conditions such as heart disease and osteoporosis. We know that before menopause women are at a lower risk of heart disease compared to our male counterparts. However, as we age, the risk increases and becomes equal for men and women. This is linked to declining oestrogen as it plays such a protective role against heart disease. Oestrogen also helps control your cholesterol levels, reducing the risk of fat building up in your arteries and keeping your blood vessels healthy. Don't be surprised if your doctor also starts to mention your blood pressure is a bit high, as this can be impacted by fluctuating hormone levels.

You've likely heard of osteoporosis, a condition of fragile bones that usually develops in later life. During perimenopause, as oestrogen falls, you begin losing bone faster than you can replace it which increases the risk. Oestrogen also helps promote calcium absorption, which builds strong bones. While you may be thinking of bone health as a 'later life' problem, it's important to stay physically strong to support your bones and muscles. Weak bones and muscles lead to bones easily breaking in your post-menopause phase, and is not something you want as you get older.

DID YOU KNOW?

Thyroid disorders are incredibly common in women, and many are unaware. Thyroid hormone disturbances, especially hypothyroidism – an underactive thyroid – may amplify and worsen the symptoms of perimenopause. Changes in oestrogen levels may lead to alterations in thyroid hormone levels, affecting metabolism, energy levels and overall health.

Why does nothing seem to help?

We have just glimpsed through the window of what is happening in your body during perimenopause. And it is a lot to digest. But please stick with me.

After clients share a myriad of symptoms, our next conversation often looks like this:

> **Client:** I have literally tried EVERYTHING. I've done detoxes, fasting diets, keto, superfood shakes, supplements, herbs, yoga... You name it, I've done it.
>
> **Sarah:** And of all those things, what, if any, made a noticeable difference?
>
> **Client:** I can honestly say I feel the same. Nothing helps and I am beginning to lose hope that any magic remedies exist.

In my experience, there are a few key reasons why nothing seems to work. The first is related to overwhelm. Overwhelm of the mind and body. If you throw eight different solutions at the problem at the same time, how do you know what, if any, are actually helping? Then, most times, the remedies, diet plans and potions become all too much, so you probably stop taking them, forget to use them or go back to Instagram to find something else. Despite all of this, you still feel exhausted and wake up in a pool of sweat at night. The impact of social media in creating a sense of overwhelm cannot be ignored here. Alarming research found that 44.7 percent of nutrition-related posts on Instagram contained inaccurate information. This study examined popular Australian accounts with over 100,000 followers that focused on nutrition. Providing some comfort, posts from dietitians and nutritionists were more accurate and of higher quality.

Worryingly, lower-quality content tended to attract more engagement.

The second key reason is related to the foundations of health. Just like the foundations of a house, you must build a solid base when it comes to your health and wellbeing. Without the right foundations, a house cannot be sturdy, long-lasting and able to withstand all kinds of weather and heavy usage. If these foundations are not absolutely solid, then the house will show defects, and may even start to fall apart. I find that many people jump to the quickest and shiniest solution when it comes to health. *What pill can I take to lose weight fast? What trend can I follow that will cure all my ails?* Society has conditioned us to chase fast fixes, and with a constant stream of content coming at us, resisting the lure of the latest health craze is not easy. What's clear is that hormonal changes in perimenopause are changing the way your body operates, so just as you adapt to other changes in life, you can adapt to support this transition.

So, I hear you ask, what is the solution?

Transforming your health is like baking a cake.

It takes multiple ingredients and the right processes to come together when making a well-structured delicious cake. Flour provides structural integrity and is absolutely essential for any cake. Then you add eggs, butter and milk to create stability, and sugar and baking powder to boost taste and texture. Optional extras come in now, depending on the type of cake. For example, fruits, nuts, chocolate and more. And finally, some cakes have icing. Not all need it, but let's be honest, most taste better with it.

Here's where the underpinning framework of your perimenopause Action Plan comes in. This process mirrors the one I take clients through in my clinical practice, where I have seen many women successfully turn around their health.

Together, we will make changes across:

YOUR NUTRITION – Just like the essential ingredient, flour, nutritional tactics and tools are absolutely critical to building a solid foundation for alleviating symptoms and supporting your body in this transition.

YOUR LIFESTYLE – Tweaks to your daily habits when it comes to sleep, stress and self-care are the eggs, butter and milk of your cake recipe. Lifestyle tactics help bolster your nutritional foundations and ensure they are fit for purpose.

YOUR SUPPLEMENTS – These optional extras can help boost an already solid foundation but are not needed in all cases. Not all cakes need choc chips, but they often go down better with them included.

YOUR MEDICATED TREATMENTS – Icing is akin to Hormone Replacement Therapy (HRT), now known as Menopausal Hormone Therapy (MHT), suitable and very effective for many women. Icing is what makes the cake taste better and if you had the option, you'd probably choose it over a plain cake, right? And it is an option, as some people can't eat icing or react poorly to it.

All of these are considerations to take into account when planning your cake recipe. Everyone's cake ingredients will be different, with mixed varieties of flour and sugar, various flavour boosters, icing and other toppers. Like cakes, no two people are the same. So, you need to find the perfect blend of tactics across nutrition, lifestyle, supplements and other treatments to improve your symptoms. If you want a better cake, you have to look at each ingredient and process and see what needs to be tweaked.

Introducing your
PERIMENOPAUSE ACTION PLAN

PLAN
Self-assessment quiz
Set goals

PREPARE
Nail your nutrition
Level up your lifestyle
Demystify supplements

DO
Create an action plan
Reflect and repeat

WHAT IS PERIMENOPAUSE?

Where do I even start? Countless women have asked me this question, especially after telling me about all the new symptoms that feel as though they popped up overnight. Major changes to your health and body can seem overwhelming. The best advice I can give you is to start with a blank page. My challenge to you is to try to forget all the noise, the advertising and the random advice from people you know, or don't, and even celebrity influencers. This is about you. This is about your journey. What worked for Claire from Pilates will not necessarily work for you.

PLAN — In the spirit of starting with a new slate, the first step in Chapter 2 is for you to complete a self-assessment quiz. It will help you clearly see what is most bothersome so you can start to realistically plan a pathway to better health and vitality. In the following pages of Chapter 2, I will guide you through a simple process to create one or two well-defined goals. Research shows that when you set a goal and write it down, you are more likely to achieve it. Structured goals help to trigger new behaviours and laser your focus on what's important to you.

PREPARE — Like anything in life, preparation is the key to success. In Chapter 3, we prepare for the nutritional tactics you will employ in your Action Plan. This includes completing a pantry and fridge reset. Trust me, it probably sounds scarier than it actually is. And I'm certainly not here to judge what's currently stocked in your home right now. This is about setting yourself up for midlife success. You will learn how to nail your nutrition with easy tactics to help with things like weight control, brain fog and hormonal symptoms. You will then focus on levelling up your lifestyle to support all areas of health, especially those where you need some extra support. And finally, I'll completely demystify the world of supplements. Not only will you become the master of recognising smart marketing tactics, you will also learn all about the top supplements I recommend, the science, the cautions and the expected results. Along the way, we will also discuss HRT and I'll leave you with key pointers for a discussion with your doctor if you need some help.

DO – This is where the rubber hits the road. Time to follow my guidance and pull together your Action Plan. After taking 3-6 months to implement changes, you can repeat the process and reset any goals that may have evolved over that time.

The small print

This book is designed to empower you with the tools and tactics you need to manage the symptoms of perimenopause. Having said that, when it comes to health and wellness, it probably won't be a surprise that not everyone stays the course. The changes you implement are designed to help you in the long term, well beyond the time you spend reading this book. Throughout the processes, I arm you with tips for sustained success, so if you detour off, you have the tools to come back on course. It is possible to change. Your journey is unique and special, just like you. I can guide you, but I cannot take the steps for you. What I can promise is to provide science-based tactics to help you manage perimenopause symptoms and get your bounce back. This journey is yours to take. It's time to put yourself first (and not feel selfish about it) so you can find the new best version of you.

By committing to this process, you are putting you first. You must fit your oxygen mask before you attend to others. Taking this journey one step at a time, setting realistic goals and sticking to your guns will pay off. Are you ready?

Clinical case: Raquel's revelation

*All case studies are based on real client experiences. Names and personal details have been changed for privacy.

Raquel, aged 41 and a project manager, came to me for help to boost her energy levels. She wanted to 'feel better' and was not sure where to turn after her recent doctor's appointment where she was told she was 'on the way to pre-diabetes'. This left her feeling frazzled. Raquel was not really sure what that meant. At her initial consultation, Raquel also mentioned her frustrations around recent weight gain, especially around her midline, despite eating healthily, going to a personal trainer twice a week and walking for at least 45 minutes every other day.

At our initial consultation, a few main clues emerged to help unlock the keys to success for Raquel:

- Raquel was under-fuelling. In a bid to lose the weight she had recently gained, she was skipping breakfast most days and eating chicken or tuna salad most nights. Several times a week, she would then snack on chocolate, cheese and crackers after dinner to satisfy her hunger cravings.

- She complained of feeling hot and sweaty most of the time, and getting more tired and cranky, particularly with her co-workers. Of much concern was waking with night sweats at least twice a week, leaving her feeling less than rested the day after.

- Her period was irregular. Some months it did not come at all.

- The only thing that seemed to boost her energy was sugar treats that provided a 'pick me up' even though an energy crash soon followed.

- A recent blood test with her doctor showed some signs of pre-diabetes. Her mother and grandmother both had type-2 diabetes which was diagnosed in their 40s.

- Raquel was taking a range of vitamins and supplements that she had researched online. Some of these had doubled-up ingredients and were not indicated for her specific concerns.

Working through my process, a new baseline was set for Raquel. Together we re-evaluated her health goals and implemented a new dietary plan. This included foods and drinks to help balance hormones and alleviate symptoms. We focused on elevating protein intake, eating to balance blood sugars and supercharging her energy levels through a range of lifestyle and mindfulness interventions. We refined her supplement regime and started two targeted supplements to assist with specific health concerns.

We worked together for just under 12 months, at which stage Raquel felt confident she had the tactics and tools to go on her own way. She experienced the following results in that time:

- 5 kg weight loss.

- Daily energy levels went from a 3 to an 8.

- Two supplements remain as part of a simplified regime.

- Blood sugar results (via repeat blood tests) showed positive trends.

- Felt empowered and confident to thrive through perimenopause.

Chapter 2
ASSESS YOURSELF AND SET CLEAR GOALS

• • • • • • • • • • • • •

SOPHIA sits at her desk and considers a nap on the corner couch. She shakes her head, rubs her eyes and yawns for what feels like the 100th time that day. She remembers what her meditation teacher covered last week in the *Introduction to Relaxation* course, held at the local library. A body scan. Yes, she needs to do that to liven up each part of her body so she has some zing for the rest of the day. There are four more candidates to interview for the General Manager position, so she has to look the part.

Sophia closes her eyes and starts with her feet. How do they feel? Today they are a bit achy, especially after she decided to do an online cardio workout this morning. Then she scans her legs. They feel tired and heavy. She's so glad she wore flats today. Moving upwards, she reaches her belly and waistline. Quite frankly, the only word she can find to describe how she feels is 'sluggish'. And then there is the pressure from her pants. She really has no idea how to shift this midline weight. Maybe it will just be this way forever?

She scans her chest area. It feels a bit tight right now as she thinks about all her symptoms. She cannot seem to quite catch her breath for a moment. Eventually, she manages to gulp down some air. She feels heavy, and her shoulders crouch over as she ponders how she can continue to go about her day feeling so average. Shoulders back and down. Breathe into it like at meditation class. Let it all go.

Finally, her head. Well, she is definitely feeling sleepy, but that is the norm lately, especially when hot sweats wake her during the night. Earlier today, she forgot her words in the middle of a sentence. She feels 'foggy'. But Sophia must admit that her mood has been pretty stable today, a nice change from yesterday when she was up and down like a yo-yo.

Deep breath. She decides today is the day. Time to find an expert to help her feel herself again. Whatever happened to the results of that DUTCH test she did a few months ago? Sophia opens her eyes and feels somewhat lighter. Taking a few moments to herself did help. The time for change is now.

• • • • • • • • • • • • •

No doubt you have found yourself in Sophia's position before. New symptoms seem to appear each week, and there isn't any consistency. From brain fog to period pain and all the aches and pains in between, your body feels different. You might feel helpless. And mind you, all this is happening while life is still plodding along in the background. Knowing how to overcome the symptoms of perimenopause seems impossible at times. In my experience, as easy as it sounds, the best place to start is at zero. Always anchor back to the knowledge that you are unique, and your symptoms and stages of perimenopause look very different to the next person.

From the start line

Step 1 in the process is to analyse your current symptoms, allowing a bigger picture view of where you are at. The easiest way to do this is to complete the self-assessment quiz. Just like Sophia's body scan, this helps you become more aware of what your body is telling you. A self-assessment also acts as a good reference point in time. Once you have completed one round of creating your perimenopause Action Plan, you may come back to it and focus on new symptoms as you progress from very early to late perimenopause. It can also help you reflect on what changes you made, and how some symptoms may no longer be as troublesome as they once were.

Your self-assessment quiz includes 'key questions' I ask women who come to me for consultations. What I love about this being a self-led process is that you only have to be honest with yourself. I have found over many years in this industry that people often feel embarrassed about some areas of their health. This means they might hold back or only tell me parts of their story. Be honest with your responses and use them as a launchpad for creating change that will be meaningful.

Following your assessment, I will guide you to create goals for your journey. SMART goals that are **S**pecific, **M**easurable, **A**ctionable, **R**ealistic and **T**imely. Well-defined goals help trigger new behaviours and focus on what's important to you. I say goals here very carefully, as you don't want to set so many goals that you feel totally overwhelmed. Research shows that when goals are documented, people are more likely to achieve them by 42 percent.

Although this step can often look arduous (and we all want to skip to the main event, right?), it's absolutely essential before you begin. In this section, you will discover what's really important when it comes to your health. From that, you will be able to devise one or two goals to help laser your focus. With set goals, you can then choose the right tips and tactics contained in this book to help transform your health.

Action Step
PERIMENOPAUSE SELF-ASSESSMENT QUIZ

A self-led questionnaire helps identify your most troublesome symptoms and assess patterns of change. When completing these questions, focus on changes that have occurred in the past 3-6 months and your most common symptoms – the ones that probably made you read this book. Take some time now to complete the quiz.

You can write in this book or use the template available at www.thenutritionpharmacist.com/book-bonuses.

If you prefer to keep your answers for comparison over time, consider printing the template or filling it out on your preferred device. Remember that you will likely come back to this quiz at a later stage, so using a template version is a good idea. That way you can save them along the way for comparison and reflection.

This quiz is not designed to be a diagnostic tool. It is a simple screening questionnaire that may indicate you are experiencing some symptoms of hormonal change. Your doctor or other medical professional is the only person who can diagnose you with perimenopause. The questions are designed for women in their perimenopause phase, but of course, it could be possible that you have transitioned to post-menopause. More reasons why this is a guide only and you need to seek appropriate medical advice.

> **Access your self-assessment quiz at**
> www.thenutritionpharmacist.com/book-bonuses
> **plus extra tools to guide you further.**

ASSESS YOURSELF AND SET CLEAR GOALS

1. Have you experienced weight gain particularly around your abdomen (aka stubborn belly fat)?
   A. No, my weight is stable.
   B. Yes, I've put on a little weight, but not enough to raise any alarms.
   C. Yes, and it seems to be impossible to lose.

2. How would you describe your daily energy levels?
   A. I feel as energetic as I always have.
   B. I feel a bit more tired than usual (more than the expected 3 pm slump).
   C. I am exhausted and feel drained by the end of the day (yay for nanna naps!).

3. Have you experienced any changes in your sleep patterns?
   A. Not at all, I sleep like a baby.
   B. Yes, I have some trouble falling asleep and/or staying asleep.
   C. Yes, I wake up many times in the night and sleep badly (hello night sweats).

4. Have you noticed changes in your mood?
   A. No, my mood seems to be stable.
   B. Yes, every now and then I have mood swings from one extreme to another.
   C. Yes, my mood changes regularly and I feel more emotional and shorter-fused than usual.

5. Are you experiencing hot flushes and/or night sweats?
   A. No, not at this stage, thankfully.
   B. Yes, on occasion, but they only seem to be mild right now.
   C. Yes, they seem to be getting worse and are really bothering me.

6. How would you rate your memory and focus?
   A. All good here, no changes.
   B. Every now and then I forget words mid-sentence or feel a bit scattered.
   C. I feel like I get brain fog almost daily and forget things quite a lot.

7. How about your menstrual cycle?
   A. It is still as regular as clockwork.
   B. My cycle is a bit irregular but not always, my flow is changing month to month and/or I have more period pain.
   C. My periods are definitely further apart, the flow is inconsistent and/or I have more period pain

8. How are your daily stress levels?
   A. About the same as they always have been.
   B. Maybe a little worse.
   C. Steadily increasing over time, I really need to do something about it.

9. Have you noticed any new or worsening aches and pains?
   A. A. No, this is not a problem for me.
   B. Yes, I especially notice it if I do more exercise or movement.
   C. Yes, I regularly experience joint and muscle aches and pains.

10. Has your libido changed?
    A. Not that I have noticed.
    B. Yes, but only a slight change from normal.
    C. Yes, I have definitely experienced lower libido than usual.

QUIZ RESULTS

Mostly As

You don't seem to be experiencing many (if any) symptoms of perimenopause. But hey, you must be here for a reason that is not included in this questionnaire. There are so many possible symptoms when it comes to perimenopause, and just because they are not listed in this short quiz, does not mean they are not important. Chances are, you are likely at the very early stages of perimenopause or have not yet entered this zone. Or there's also the chance you may be managing your symptoms well already. List your main areas of concern here to help you when it comes to developing SMART goals, e.g. dizziness, dry skin.

_____

_____

_____

Mostly Bs

You seem to be experiencing some classic signs of perimenopause. Based on your responses, your symptoms are typical of the earlier stages of perimenopause and appear milder. The good news? In this zone, you are most likely to see greater benefits from diet and lifestyle changes. There is also the possibility you are in later stages, but managing some of your symptoms already. Below, list the top one or two symptoms that are causing you the most daily disturbance to help you to create SMART goals, e.g. cannot lose belly fat, always tired.

_____

_____

_____

Mostly Cs

Your body is going through some significant changes. Based on your responses, your symptoms seem more like the later phases of perimenopause. The good news is that diet and lifestyle changes, coupled with other supportive treatments, will be helpful. For now, focus on the one to two symptoms causing you the most discomfort and list these below. This will help form your SMART goals, e.g. low libido, brain fog, hot flushes.

_____

_____

_____

How do you get a diagnosis of perimenopause?

When it comes to getting a perimenopause diagnosis, this one is a little cloudy so to speak. While there is no one blood test to diagnose perimenopause, there are some options at your disposal. As described in Chapter 1, your oestrogen levels will fluctuate from highs to lows on a regular basis. As such, any blood test will only show a snapshot of what is happening on that particular day and time. Once you progress to menopause, blood tests may be more helpful. This is a big bugbear for women, and a common complaint I've heard when it comes to receiving care. 'I went to the doctor and they said there is no test. They said I must be really busy which causes fatigue, or maybe I am heading to perimenopause.' Unfortunately, blood tests are not overly helpful in formalising a diagnosis. However, it's not to say they are never valuable. Blood tests to investigate your hormone levels may be helpful in showing general trends over time or if you want to see how HRT is changing levels in your body. Timing is important when it comes to hormonal blood tests, as a key marker of ovulation is the level of progesterone. If you have ovulated, levels of progesterone usually peak around day 21 of your cycle, indicating an egg has been released. This is why you usually have hormone-related blood tests 7 days before your next period.

So how do you get diagnosed?

The greatest predictors of the perimenopause transition are your symptoms. Your best bet is to keep track of symptoms, so you can show your doctor how they progress over time to get a gauge of what stage of perimenopause you may be in.

> **Download your perimenopause symptom checklist at** www.thenutritionpharmacist.com/book-bonuses
> **plus extra tools to guide you further.**

Action Step
PERIMENOPAUSE SYMPTOM CHECKLIST

Make a note of any of these symptoms in your diary every few days or when you remember. Keeping track can show how things may be changing over time. Show these trends to your doctor or other health professional, so they can review and determine what your best treatment, diet and lifestyle options are.

YOUR CYCLE

- ☐ Less frequent periods
- ☐ Lighter or heavier periods
- ☐ Irregular periods
- ☐ Spotting between cycles
- ☐ Period cramps and/or pain

YOUR MOOD AND FOCUS

- ☐ Low mood
- ☐ Mood swings
- ☐ Anxiety
- ☐ Irritability
- ☐ Brain fog
- ☐ Poor concentration and/or memory
- ☐ More forgetful than usual

OTHER SYMPTOMS

- ☐ Breast pain and/or tenderness
- ☐ Headaches
- ☐ Midline weight gain
- ☐ Weight gain in general
- ☐ Low libido
- ☐ Fatigue
- ☐ Trouble sleeping
- ☐ Hot flushes
- ☐ Night sweats
- ☐ Vaginal dryness
- ☐ Dry skin
- ☐ Fluid retention
- ☐ Joint aches and/or pains
- ☐ Frozen shoulder
- ☐ Dizziness
- ☐ Tinnitus

ASSESS YOURSELF AND SET CLEAR GOALS

Use this space to list other symptoms you may experience:

General bloodwork is helpful

Don't forget your annual blood test!

Stay curious when it comes to your health and speak to your doctor about an annual blood test to identify any specific areas that need attention. There could quite possibly be other reasons for your symptoms. Don't simply assume it is perimenopause. Let me give you a common example. You can implement all the known tactics to boost your energy levels, from eating energy-boosting foods, cutting down on coffee and getting more sleep. But if you have low levels of iron or your thyroid function is not optimal, this will continue to impact your energy levels. Having a blood test and then rectifying any deficiencies or areas of concern means you are starting from a level playing field. Here are some blood tests to discuss with your doctor during perimenopause.

A full blood count (FBC) and comprehensive metabolic panel (CMP)

Looks at things like red blood cells, white blood cells and platelets. CMP reveals information about your overall metabolism, including kidney and liver function, and electrolytes such as sodium and potassium which can show how well hydrated (or dehydrated) you might be.

Lipid profile

This checks your total cholesterol, HDL ('good') cholesterol, LDL ('bad') cholesterol and triglycerides. Declining oestrogen can mean your cholesterol levels are less well controlled, placing you at higher risk of heart health changes over time.

Diabetes tests, fasting blood glucose and HbA1c

These tests look for signs of insulin resistance which can become an issue for some women.

Nutritional deficiencies, e.g. vitamin D, zinc, vitamin B12 and magnesium

Symptoms such as fatigue, poor immune health and mood disorders may be related to low levels of these important nutrients. When it comes to magnesium, bear in mind that this blood test is not overly accurate. Less than 1 percent of total body magnesium is present in the blood, so a magnesium blood test may not truly reflect total body magnesium levels but can be used as a guide.

Iron studies, e.g. iron, ferritin, transferrin

Many symptoms of perimenopause mirror those of low iron, or iron deficiency, e.g. brain fog, low energy levels and dizziness. You will find out why iron is so important in Chapter 3.

Thyroid function tests, e.g. TSH, free T4, free T3, reverse T3, anti-TPO and anti-thyroglobulin

These tests are a good screening tool for any thyroid conditions which may cause perimenopause-type symptoms (e.g. weight gain, fatigue, forgetfulness).

DUTCH hormone test

This is a test commonly recommended by some practitioners. Unfortunately, the same theory applies here. The DUTCH test (Dried Urine Test for Comprehensive Hormones) has the same limitations at this stage of change. It will only capture a moment in time which is varying significantly in perimenopause. If you want to capture hormonal trends over time, just like blood tests, these may be useful but will not provide an absolute diagnosis of your stage of perimenopause.

Action Step
SMART GOALS

S is for specific. A goal linked to one activity, thought, or idea.
M is for measurable. A goal you can track and measure progress towards.
A is for actionable. Clear tasks or actions you can take to make progress toward a goal.
R is for realistic.
T is for timely.

Begin with your top one or two most troubling symptoms to help zone in on the action steps. As you implement new tactics to manage these symptoms, you will find that other areas of your health and wellbeing thrive at the same time.

Here is an example as a guide:

Goal: I want to lose 10 kg of body weight in the next 6 months by using tactics and tools in my perimenopause Action Plan.
Top concerns: address stubborn belly fat, gained weight cannot shift.

Goal: I want to rate my energy levels as an 8 out of 10 (*10 being my best ever energy level) 3 months from today by following my Action Plan.
Top concerns: drop in energy levels, fatigue, brain fog.

Goal: I want to rate my hormonal symptoms as less than 3 out of 10 (currently 7 out of 10) in 3 months using the science-backed tactics I discovered in this book.
Top concerns: hot flushes, night sweats, mood swings, brain fog.

ASSESS YOURSELF AND SET CLEAR GOALS

Be clear about your goals and write them down

Goal:

___

___

___

Top concerns:

___

___

___

Goal:

___

___

___

Top concerns:

___

___

___

Goal:

Top concerns:

Where to from here?

You have set your SMART goals. Firstly, take a moment to thank yourself for doing this. Now, think of these goals as your visualisations of desired outcomes when it comes to this transformative journey. As you move to Part II of this book, the true magic happens.

While it's awesome to have set goals, one limitation of SMART goals is that they do not specify 'how' the goal will be achieved. In Part II, we learn all about the 'how' so you have the key tactics and tools across nutrition, lifestyle, supplements and other treatments to help you work towards your goals each and every day. See you there.

Clinical case: Danielle's discovery

All case studies are based on real client experiences. Names and personal details have been changed for privacy.

Danielle's story is one I come across all too often. Being a nutritionist, I find it is common for clients to see me as a weight-loss guru, and often only that.

Danielle, aged 38, came to me with a real concern about her midlife weight gain. In her words, she was 'hovering' around 8 kg above her goal weight, the weight she used to be a good few years ago. None of her old clothes fit her anymore and she honestly felt this all stemmed back to the COVID pandemic. She believed she had gained weight due to all the Melbourne lockdowns and it never really shifted. Danielle was very clear on what she wanted to get out of our time together. She wanted help to reset her diet with a meal plan, so she knew exactly what to do when and could avoid all temptation. She wanted a strict approach, as she claimed to have zero willpower.

At our initial one-hour appointment, we went through a variety of questions, including the themes covered in the self-assessment quiz. Here's what we uncovered:

- Danielle often used food as a pick-me-up. She was experiencing energy highs and lows, leaving her feeling rock-bottom exhausted at least three times a week.

- She had no real 'downtime'. Danielle had a demanding job where she worked almost six days a week. This left little time to unwind and relax.

- Of late, she noticed small things annoying her (almost) daily, leading to mood swings and her being more snappy with family.

- The two things she found most frustrating were her midline weight gain and constantly feeling on edge and anxious.

ASSESS YOURSELF AND SET CLEAR GOALS

When I came back to Danielle with her next steps following our initial appointment, I held back from devising a meal plan (more on why I do not think these are a great long-term tool later!). In her follow-up notes and action plan, I played back the summary of her symptoms as I heard them, and noted she seemed to have more concerns than her weight in isolation. I suggested we work together to create SMART goals so we could create a focus point, and I could build a diet, lifestyle and supplement plan around that for her.

With her agreement, here is where we landed:

Danielle: I want to lose 3 kg of body weight in the next 6 months by implementing diet and lifestyle changes recommended by my nutritionist.

Sarah: Break it down. Specific: body weight. Measurable: 3 kg. Achievable and realistic: half-a-kilo per month. Time-bound: 6 months.

Danielle: I want to feel more in control of my moods 6 months from today (experiencing mood swings once a week or less), using tactics across nutrition, lifestyle and supplements, as recommended by my nutritionist.

Sarah: Break it down. Specific: mood changes. Measurable: from almost daily to once or less a week. Achievable and realistic: reducing frequency versus complete elimination. Time-bound: 6 months.

The discovery here for Danielle was that she was placing too much emphasis on her weight alone. Our consultation helped her realise she was experiencing a raft of symptoms, and that all of them together were likely contributing to her feeling pretty down on herself at this stage of life. Working through a holistic assessment helps to draw out what matters most, setting clients like Danielle – and you – up for the best success.

Part II
SCIENCE-BASED SOLUTIONS

Now that we've established the foundations, assessed your symptoms and set SMART goals, it's time to learn what you can do to feel like you again. I've found there are three key areas to focus on when it comes to managing symptoms of perimenopause:

1. Nutrition
2. Lifestyle
3. Supplements

Then there are medical treatments to discuss with your doctor. While there is a lot to unpack in each of these areas, I'm focusing on tactics and tools my clients have had success with, those that are relatively easy to implement and only with science to back them up.

My suggestion is to read through this section entirely first. Let it all sink in and think about how relevant each part is to your life. Armed with all this information, we will then move into Chapter 6 where it will all come together.

PLAN

Self-assessment quiz
Set goals

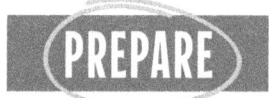

PREPARE

Nail your nutrition
Level up your lifestyle
Demystify supplements

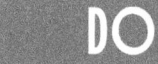

DO

Create an action plan
Reflect and repeat

Chapter 3
NUTRITION TOOLS AND TACTICS

• • • • • • • • • • • • •

6:30 am Pilates class. It seemed like a good idea when Sophia booked it last week. What is it they say? Win the morning, win the day? She lies back, closes her eyes and enjoys a few moments of rest on her reformer. Sophia can't help overhearing a conversation between two ladies in the front row.

'You look amazing, Liz! What's the secret?'

Liz declares she has eliminated carbs on what she calls a semi-keto diet. She seriously thinks this is the best diet she has ever tried. She learnt about it from her sister who lost a lot of weight using this method.

'Oh yes, I'm about to start a new diet,' says Catherine, as she nods her head in deep agreement with Liz. 'I've found one that will not only help me slim down, but also removes any toxins from my blood stream which reduces this daily brain fog I'm having. I feel like I would do anything to make it go away!'

Sophia wonders what she's missed here. She hasn't considered a keto diet before. She makes a mental note to Google it when she gets home. I mean, she is about to start working on reaching these new health goals soon, and she should probably stay on track with that. But these ladies might be on to something new. And they even said it eliminates brain fog! If it works for them, it has to work for her.

'Time to get started. Set your springs on a blue-yellow for intermediate, and a blue-red for my advanced ladies.'

Time to get moving. As the class begins, a wash of thoughts pass through Sophia's mind. *Surely this nutrition thing can't be that hard.* Sophia shakes her head and takes a deep breath in and out through her mouth like blowing through a straw.

• • • • • • • • • • • • •

Changing health behaviours is hard. It's often made harder by some of the simplest things, like following advice from well-meaning acquaintances. The good news is that making changes to your nutrition in perimenopause might be easier than you think. Nutrition is the flour to your cake. It provides structural integrity and is a vital foundation for true health. Adapting your nutrition with science-based tactics can ensure your foundations are as solid as possible.

What I love about making dietary changes is that it's one of those things you can change and actually notice a difference. Some benefits can happen quickly, others amplify in the long term, but one thing's for sure. These changes help all areas of health and kickstart your journey to better managing symptoms.

However, I'm sure you'll agree that just like Sophia, you can't help but overhear the chatter about what has worked for others or what new nutrition trend is on the horizon. It has to be one of the most confusing, overwhelming and controversial topics. Everyone seems to have an opinion on what's healthy, what's not and how they achieved amazing results using a proven method or a new fad diet. I'm here to assure you it doesn't have to be hard.

Nutrition and perimenopause

Simply put, hormonal changes in perimenopause alter the way your body operates. So, it only makes sense that you need to adapt your nutrition to help best navigate these changes. Your body continues to need key nutrients to stay healthy, but it needs more of some things and less of others. Let's walk through my top science-backed nutrition tactics for perimenopause. For now, take the time to review the content and think about how it is relevant to your diet. You will develop your Action Plan, choosing the tactics that best support achieving your SMART goals.

9 top nutrition tactics FOR PERIMENOPAUSE

Tactic 1

LEVEL UP YOUR PROTEIN

IN A NUTSHELL: Ensure you have enough protein on your plate, especially at breakfast, and spread evenly throughout the day.

HELPS WITH: Weight control, muscle growth and maintenance, blood sugar control.

To start, let's discuss a non-negotiable when it comes to adding new tactics to your diet. Clients tell me that keeping an eye on their protein intake feels like a part-time job. But there are so many reasons why it's worth the effort. Protein is a valuable nutrient at all stages of life, but even more so for women in perimenopause. Here's why:

- You naturally lose more muscle with age, which leads to an increased appetite for protein. In other words, if you don't meet your daily protein targets, you can be left overconsuming other potentially less nutritious foods as your body tries to drive increased protein intake.

- Protein helps keep you fuller for longer. If you always feel hungry, or just don't seem satisfied after meals, consider how much protein you are including. Protein suppresses the hormone called ghrelin to stimulate a feeling of fullness. Eating sufficient protein in perimenopause keeps you feeling satisfied as well as supporting muscle health and mitigating muscle loss.

- Protein helps keep your blood sugars in check. By slowing the absorption of glucose into your bloodstream, sufficient protein helps your body regulate blood sugar levels. This promotes a gradual release of glucose into the bloodstream, supporting any insulin resistance that may be contributing to weight gain.

So, how much protein do you actually need during perimenopause? Ideally, you should aim for 1-1.2 grams of protein per kilogram of body weight per day. Some research also suggests ranges of 1.4-2.2 g/kg which is at the higher end for more active women. I like to start with the 1-1.2 gram recommendation, as even this can be a lot to pack in. Spreading protein across the day is important, and a higher amount at breakfast is best to support muscle growth.

Here's a rough guide, which varies based on your weight:

Breakfast: aim for 20–30 grams. This should be your most protein-rich meal of the day.

Lunch and dinner: aim for at least 20-30 grams.

Snacks: add protein to top up your intake throughout the day, as you may not always reach targets at main meals.

> **You'll find protein-rich recipe ideas at**
> **@the_nutrition_pharmacist**

Food and drink protein sources

Here is a quick reference guide to some common protein-rich foods. Where possible, check product nutrition labels as amounts will vary based on the brand you use.

Protein source	Amount	Approximate level of protein
Cottage cheese	100 grams	12 grams
Hard cheese	40 grams	10 grams
Greek or natural yoghurt	200 grams	10 grams
High protein yoghurt	160-170 grams	15 grams
Dairy milk	1 cup	8-9 grams
Soy milk	1 cup	7-8 grams
Oat milk	1 cup	1-4 grams
Almond milk	1 cup	1-2 grams
Beef, chicken, lamb, pork	100 grams cooked/lean	30 grams
Fish fillets	100 grams cooked	25 grams
Canned tuna	95 gram can	18 grams
Egg	1 medium egg	6 grams
Tofu	100 grams	10 grams
Tempeh	100 grams	10–15 grams
Chickpeas, lentils, red kidney beans	½ cup (canned)	5 grams
Edamame	½ cup cooked (fresh or frozen)	8 grams
Peanut butter	1 tablespoon	6 grams
Protein powders	Serve size as per packaging information	20-25 grams depending on brand
Hemp seeds	1 tablespoon	3 grams

Sunflower seeds	1 tablespoon	2 grams
Chia seeds	1 tablespoon	3 grams
Protein pasta	½ cup cooked	6 grams (very brand dependent)
Rolled oats	½ cup dry	5 grams

Provides a guide only. Individual products vary.

My thoughts on protein powders

Personally, I find protein powders make it easier to meet protein targets, especially on busy days. Adding a few scoops to yoghurt or smoothies is my go-to for breakfast and snacks. You don't necessarily need protein powder, but if you like them and they make your life easier, I say, why not. Choose a product with minimal additives and give a few brands a go to see what you tolerate best. You may hear chatter about these powders being highly 'processed'. Yes, they undergo processing, which is common for many food products. Other protein sources like tofu, meat products and cheeses also undergo some processing. It's what makes food edible and palatable in some instances. How could we eat bread if we did not mill and grind wheat to flour? The unprocessed form is inedible! Yes, protein powders typically undergo more processing than other food sources of protein. So, you may like to choose whole foods where you can. But protein powders may be convenient on some occasions. It all comes down to balance.

Guidance on the different types of protein powders

Whey protein, derived from dairy milk, is the most common type of protein found in powders, and is easily digested by your body. Whey is very effective when it comes to increasing the production of new protein in muscles, particularly when consumed close to exercise. When it comes to whey, you may notice the words isolate, concentrate or hydrolysate on the label. What does this mean? It simply comes down to how the product is processed and the amount of protein, fat, carbohydrate and lactose in each serve. At the end of the day, all formats have pretty similar evidence of benefits.

Whey concentrate is less processed than isolate, but contains less protein and more fats, carbs and lactose per serve.

Whey isolate is more highly processed, but has higher protein levels, less lactose per serve and may be better tolerated in cases of lactose intolerance. This form is usually more expensive.

Whey hydrolysate is the most highly processed and is designed for faster and easier absorption. It has a similar composition to the isolate form.

Casein protein, also derived from dairy milk, is often found in protein powders. Casein is more slowly absorbed than whey, but taken in the evening, it can provide a slow and steady release of amino acids, protein's building blocks, for long periods where you do not eat, like while asleep. Casein protein is not as effective as whey protein when it comes to stimulating the muscle-building processes in your body.

Protein supplements for a plant-based diet

The list below is certainly not exhaustive! However, it covers plant-based protein types commonly found in protein powders Down Under.

Soy protein

Soy protein, derived from ground soybeans, is a great high-protein plant-based option. Soy products contain phytoestrogens (more on this later) which should be avoided in some people.

Pea protein

Typically made from yellow or green peas, this is another plant-based option. Muscle-related gains have been shown to be similar to those using whey protein.

Hemp protein

From the seeds of the cannabis plant, minus the psychoactive element, hemp protein contains a moderate amount of protein as well as being a source of fibre, iron, zinc, magnesium and alpha-linolenic acid (a plant-based way to get some omega-3s).

Other plant-based proteins

You will also see rice, almond, peanut and other sources of plant protein. Each has its own touted benefits, which you can explore. Just ensure you opt for products with ingredients you are happy to consume regularly, and that the protein levels per serve are providing you the top-up you need for your day.

Tactic 2
CHOOSE SMART CARBS

IN A NUTSHELL: Choose smart carbohydrates that slowly digest, providing you with sustained energy throughout the day.

HELPS WITH: Weight control, blood sugar control, low energy levels.

When it comes to fuelling your body throughout the day, you want to fill your tank with foods that sustain energy. Ever eaten a piece of cake or fast-food burger only to find yourself in an energy slump a few hours later? This is because some foods release energy in fast doses, but don't provide long-lasting effects. Choose foods and drinks that have a low glycaemic index (GI) so energy is released gradually, providing a steady level throughout the day. These foods are often referred to as 'smart carbs'. Smart carbs keep your blood sugar levels stable throughout the day, eliminating bouts of hunger that come with those sugar lows. Here are some smart carbs for you to stock up on and include in your meals and snacks.

Bread, rolls, wraps and crisps
- Wholegrain breads, rolls, crackers or wraps
- Pumpernickel breads
- Soy and linseed breads, rolls or crackers
- Authentic sourdough
- Roti or naan bread made with chickpea flour

Pasta, noodles, rice and the like
- Wholegrain or brown basmati rice, low-GI rice, wild rice
- Pulse-based pastas (e.g. lentil pasta)
- Soba noodles
- Mung bean noodles

Breakfast options
- Traditional rolled oats or steel-cut oats
- Wheat, rice or oat bran

Veggies
- Orange sweet potato (if you like white potato, leave the skin on for a smarter carb option)
- Canned vegetables (low or no salt varieties) e.g. edamame, chickpeas, lentils, black beans (most also available in dried form)

And now for some great news! Not only are smart carbs good for your energy levels, they may also reduce the severity of hot flushes, simply by regulating your blood sugar levels. I mean, do you need any more reasons to switch?

What about intermittent fasting in perimenopause?

Intermittent fasting is where you eat between specific times and fast during others. A common method is known as 16:8, where you eat in an 8-hour window, and fast for the remaining 16 hours, e.g. eat between 12 noon and 8 pm. Studies confirm various benefits of fasting for health, such as weight loss, improved insulin sensitivity and reduced inflammation. All these benefits are potentially helpful in perimenopause. However, there is a chance that fasting may impact hormonal imbalances and/or place additional stress on the body. (Limited research exists on this in women, but one animal study suggests fasting causes changes in oestrogen levels). When it comes to fasting, I recommend speaking to your doctor or other health professionals, so you can have a personalised plan and be monitored for outcomes.

Tactic 3

CROWD YOUR PLATE WITH PLANT FOODS

IN A NUTSHELL: Pack your plate with as many plants as possible to keep you full and well nourished.

HELPS WITH: Weight control, blood sugar control, low energy levels, brain fog, heart health, gut health.

This one is all about prioritising plant foods. Fill your plate with a variety of fruits, veggies and herbs, and serve with lean proteins and smart carbs. This technique is called crowding, as it does just that. It 'crowds' or fills up your stomach with lower calorie but highly nutritious foods and leaves less 'room' for other less healthy foods. This also keeps you feeling full and satisfied after meals and prevents snacking between meals.

While this is a great way to support weight loss and weight maintenance, as well as providing your body with the key nutrients it needs to thrive, it also gives you an abundance of plant-based antioxidants that are packed with goodness. Antioxidants play a protective role in many areas of health. For example:

- Eating a variety of antioxidant-rich foods each week can boost gut health, which can in turn elevate mood. Research shows that people who eat more than thirty different plant foods per week have a more diverse collection of microbes in the gut – which is good for so many areas of your health especially immune and mental health.

- Eating the colours of the rainbow has major benefits for symptoms such as confusion and memory loss. Many studies support that flavonoids (a specific type of plant antioxidant) help improve the flow of oxygen and blood in the brain to improve brain function. A healthy brain is less susceptible to lapses in cognition, aka brain fog. To pack more flavonoids into your day, eat these foods: oranges, capsicums, celery, strawberries, apples, pears and bananas.

- Other widespread benefits of eating antioxidants include protecting heart health and balancing blood fats.

TIPS

Fruits and veggies with a purplish colour are usually higher in flavonoid antioxidants. Think blueberries, blackberries, cherries, and yes, red wine (in moderation of course!). Flavonoids also reduce inflammation in the body, which can have many benefits in perimenopause.

Spice it up with additions like turmeric, ginger and cayenne pepper which have anti-inflammatory properties, while making meals more creative and tasty!

Nuts and seeds also count as plant foods. Add them to salads for crunch or eat a palmful as a tasty snack.

To employ this tactic, eat as many different coloured plant foods that you can across your day. Vibrant colours are a sign there are plenty of antioxidants in your choice. Variety is the spice of life, and your body loves to reap the benefits from all kinds of different fresh foods, so the key is to mix it up a little. Why not try something new this week?

Love your cruciferous veggies

Have you ever heard of cruciferous vegetables? There's no doubt you've eaten your fair share. Part of the *Brassica* genus of plants, they include these common veggies: Brussels sprouts, broccoli, kale, cabbage, cauliflower, bok choy, radishes and turnips. Not only are these morsels packed with nutrients, vitamins and fibre, they also have several unique benefits:

- Cruciferous veggies contain glucosinolates, responsible for the pungent aroma and bitter flavour. When chewed and digested, glucosinolates break down to active compounds, one of which is known as sulforaphane. Sulforaphane has a range of health benefits, including acting as an antioxidant and anti-inflammatory, reducing low-grade chronic inflammation in this life era. Sulforaphane supports the body to clear excess oestrogen when levels are high.

- When you eat certain cruciferous vegetables such as broccoli, your body also makes diindolylmethane (DIM), a compound which is thought to help restore oestrogen balance. It does this by helping the liver metabolise oestrogen more effectively.

Next time you are choosing what greens to have with dinner, you have so many reasons to choose the humble broccoli.

TIP

Your liver plays a critical role in the regulation of oestrogen in the body, breaking it down for elimination. If your liver function is sluggish, this could impact oestrogen levels and hormone balance.

Tactic 4

BALANCE YOUR HORMONES WITH PHYTOESTROGENS

IN A NUTSHELL: Try adding one or two serves of phytoestrogen-rich foods to your diet each day to reap hormone-balancing benefits.

HELPS WITH: Hormonal symptoms (e.g. mood changes, brain fog, hot flushes).

As you know, oestrogen levels fluctuate in perimenopause. By including certain foods in your diet, you may be able to somewhat alleviate symptoms such as hot flushes, night sweats, low energy, brain fog, mood fluctuations and more. Phytoestrogens, found in some plants, are phytonutrients that have a similar chemical structure to oestrogen. While they are not an exact replacement for oestrogen, they are able to weakly bind to oestrogen receptors in the body. These foods work in an interesting way, either being classified as 'pro-oestrogen' or 'anti-oestrogen'. Essentially, their actions depend on the level of circulating oestrogen in the body at the time, and they work via a variety of mechanisms to help the body to achieve balance.

Mixed research suggests that Japanese women who eat a traditional phytoestrogen-rich diet, one including foods like tofu, miso and fermented or boiled soybeans, may experience fewer hot flushes than women living in Western countries.

While it sounds like these foods may be the solution to all your perimenopause problems, there are a few things to be aware of. Only around one in three women who add phytoestrogens to their diet actually see the benefits in terms of alleviating hormonal symptoms. This may be because, in the gut, phytoestrogens generally need to be converted by special bacteria to be effective. And not everyone has that gut bacteria. In addition, phytoestrogens are not very well absorbed by the body. This means to have an effect, you need to eat relatively high amounts. So, if you try adding more phytoestrogen-rich foods for a few weeks and notice no real difference, you may need to look at some other tactics.

Here are some ways to add phytoestrogens to your diet

Add some soy to your day. Isoflavones, found in soybeans, are phytoestrogens. Soy products also contain bioactive compounds called genistein and daidzein. These may help relieve hot flushes.

Food sources: Tempeh, soybeans, tofu, miso, edamame (young soybeans), soy milk and soy drinks.

A note on soy products: For some women, soy products may not be well tolerated. They may contribute to breast pain, or hamper the ability to lose body fat due to a variety of complex reasons. If you notice that soy makes your breasts more tender, or you are not shifting body weight despite other combined efforts, consider getting other sources of phytoestrogens in your diet. And speak to a qualified nutrition professional who can guide you more specifically.

Lignans please!

This type of phytoestrogen is found in flaxseeds, whole grains, legumes, fruits and veggies.

Food sources: Oats, rice, barley, quinoa, flaxseed, sesame seeds, sunflower seeds, pistachios, almonds, chickpeas, lentils, red kidney beans, broccoli and cabbage.

Other sources of phytoestrogens: Garlic, turmeric, carrots, celery, spinach, alfalfa, pomegranates and berries.

What does a serve look like?
- A glass of soy milk
- 200 grams of tofu or tempeh
- 40 grams of ground flaxseed (ground ones make it easier for

your body to absorb all the goodness)
- 2 slices of soy-linseed bread (Linseeds and flaxseeds are the same thing!)

How much should you have in your diet?

Start by including one to two serves per day for about three months and see if they improve your symptoms. You really don't have much to lose, as these are healthy, nutritious foods, even if they don't make things noticeably better.

A note on phytoestrogens and breast cancer risk

There is a common circulating message that phytoestrogens cause breast cancer. However, some evidence suggests that phytoestrogens play a protective role against breast cancer for those who have had higher levels in their diet since childhood. The caveat here is this. In people who have HER-2-positive tumours and any premenopausal women at high risk of breast cancer, **it is best to avoid them.** If this is relevant for you, please discuss with your doctor, and do not implement the tactics related to adding more phytoestrogens to your diet before you do so.

Get your phytoestrogens from the most natural sources possible, as highly processed soy products behave differently in the body and may have different effects when it comes to cancer risk.

More natural soy products include soy milk, edamame and tofu.

Processed soy products usually contain textured vegetable protein and soy protein isolate. Check soy-based protein powders and nutrition bars which may contain these ingredients.

Tactic 5

OMEGA-3S FOR BRAIN AND HEART HEALTH

IN A NUTSHELL: Add omega-3s to your plate to boost brain health, promote a healthy mood and support a healthy heart.

HELPS WITH: Brain fog, mood changes, heart and cholesterol health.

Omega-3s are a bit of an unsung hero in my book. When it comes to managing mood swings and brain fog, the inclusion of omega-3 fatty acids in your diet may just help keep your brain function and emotions in check. They do this by supporting brain cell communication as well as reducing inflammation. At the same time, omega-3s are a powerhouse for your heart health. Once menopause hits, your heart disease risk increases and your blood fats and cholesterol levels can start to go off track, amongst other things. Including omega-3s in your diet may help balance your blood fats and cholesterol, slightly reduce or stabilise blood pressure and reduce the chances of getting an irregular heartbeat (arrhythmia). We will cover more about the benefits of omega-3s in Chapter 5, when we look at supplements. Good sources of omega-3 in the diet include the following. Aim to include these in your diet at least three times a week.

- Oily fish, like anchovies, sardines, mackerel, herring, salmon, trout and swordfish.

- To get omega-3s through plant sources, you need to include foods such as walnuts, flaxseeds, chia seeds, hemp seeds, edamame and seaweed. These foods are a good source of alpha-linolenic acid which then converts to omega-3s in the body. Most plant sources do not contain EPA and DHA – the types of omega-3 fats with specific health benefits.

Tactic 6

EAT ENERGY-BOOSTING FOODS

IN A NUTSHELL: Eat foods that contain B vitamins and iron to support energy levels.

HELPS WITH: Brain fog, low energy levels.

Energy levels can fluctuate on a daily basis, and 3:30 pm 'itis' may feel even more extreme in perimenopause. B vitamins and iron are the two powerhouses when it comes to giving your body energy.

B vitamins help you release energy from food. Pack more Bs into your day by eating a wide variety of veggies, fruit, grainy breads, lean protein and dairy products. For those following a vegetarian or vegan diet, pay special attention to getting vitamin B12 which is mainly found in animal products. It can also be found in some fortified cereals, plant milks, meat substitute products, nutritional yeast, tempeh and nori seaweed.

Iron plays a key role in regulating your energy levels (amongst other things, such as supporting a healthy immune response). As a transporter of oxygen in your blood, it provides energy for daily life. Iron intake is particularly important in perimenopause, more so for women who have heavier periods which can reduce iron stores. At the same time, declining oestrogen levels may reduce iron absorption and storage in the body. Keeping up your intake of dietary iron is a good way to support a healthy balance. Iron can be found in the diet in animal sources (haem iron) and non-animal sources (non-haem iron). Haem iron is much better absorbed by the body than non-haem iron, so those following strict vegetarian or vegan diets may need to consider iron supplementation in consultation with their doctor.

Generally, if you eat a variety of foods such as meat, plants, nuts and seeds, you will get sufficient daily iron. In Australia, it is recommended that women aged 19-50 get 18 mg of iron daily, while women over 50 require 8 mg (as menstruation has usually stopped). For those on a plant-based diet, your iron needs are 1.8 times greater, as the plant sources are not as well absorbed. This equates to 32 mg for women in the perimenopause age bracket.

Haem iron: Meat, poultry, seafood and organ meats.

Non-haem iron: Nuts, seeds, legumes and tofu. Examples include mixed baked beans, lentils and chickpeas, and dark leafy green vegetables like spinach, silver beet and broccoli.

When including iron on your plate, there are some ways you can better promote its absorption. Pair iron-rich food with fruits and vegetables high in vitamin C such as citrus fruits, tomatoes, capsicums and berries. At the same time, avoid eating iron-rich foods with blockers that can make it harder for your body to absorb iron. Blockers include tea, coffee, red wine and foods rich in calcium.

Tactic 7

STAY WELL HYDRATED, AND LIMIT CAFFEINE AND ALCOHOL

IN A NUTSHELL: Be consistent with 8-10 glasses of water a day and limit alcohol and caffeine.

HELPS WITH: Weight control, brain fog, mood changes, low energy levels.

This easy tactic can have mounds of benefits. Your brain loves being well hydrated so it can stay alert and sharp. At the same time, water helps absorb all the wonderful nutrients from food so they can provide energy. No doubt you've heard that you need to aim for 8-10 glasses of water a day, which is roughly two litres. This is pretty much spot on for the most part, but in some cases, you may need more, such as in warmer weather or when you sweat more through exercise, hot flushes or night sweats. On these days, make sure you add a few extra glasses to be sure. Water is the best option, but for some this can get a tad boring. Try infusing water with citrus fruits or berries, or enjoy a refreshing iced tea. When you exercise intensely for over 60 minutes or sweat excessively, add in a glass or two of an electrolyte drink. This replaces lost salts and helps rehydrate your body faster. Making sure you drink enough water may also help keep your appetite at bay, stimulate your body's metabolism and energy expenditure, and ultimately help with weight control.

What about coffee and alcohol?

While coffee is a delightful beverage for most, caffeine is probably affecting your energy levels. Where most people go wrong with caffeine is they assume it gives them energy. In fact, all caffeine does is stop you feeling tired. It blocks a substance called adenosine from working in the brain to stop you feeling sleepy. That wears off and you are right back where you started, maybe even more tired, and looking for another hit. The body also adapts. Regular caffeine drinkers simply produce more adenosine, leaving them asking for a triple-shot latte to feel the effects. Sound familiar? If so, it might be a good idea to cut back or consider adding in some decaf. If it makes a difference for you, it could be worth the small sacrifice for the greater good! For some women, caffeine may trigger or worsen hot flushes. If this is the case for you, maybe it's best to avoid caffeine or switch to decaf, herbal tea or cooler drinks for a little while to see if this makes a material difference.

And to address the elephant in the room, alcohol is not your friend in perimenopause. It can hinder your liver function as well as mess up your energy levels. Alcohol can also impact your sleep quality. Again, for some, alcohol may worsen hot flushes. Of course, not everyone is going to eliminate this, but consider limiting your intake if you want to feel more energetic and less sluggish while keeping your hydration in check. Needless to say, if weight management is a goal, alcohol is typically high in calories and contains little nutritional value for your body. If you notice a connection, you are best to limit your intake.

NUTRITION TOOLS AND TACTICS

Tactic 8
NOURISH YOUR GUT HEALTH

IN A NUTSHELL: Include gut-nourishing foods such as whole foods, fermented foods, prebiotics and probiotics.

HELPS WITH: Weight control, low energy levels, mood changes, brain fog.

What's going on in your gut can impact many areas of the body. Keeping your bowel movements regular and managing stomach symptoms is one reason to ensure you nourish your gut with the right food and drinks. What may not be so obvious are the benefits of a healthy gut when it comes to your perimenopause symptoms. Did you know that a healthy gut microbiome – the collection of bacteria and other micro-organisms in your gut – has the ability to positively impact your mood, energy levels and overall mental health and weight? In fact, in science, the gut has been called the second brain because it can make the same chemical messengers (e.g. serotonin, dopamine) as the brain does, and these are responsible for regulating pleasure, reward and emotions. And when it comes to weight control, certain strains of gut healthy probiotics have been linked with controlling appetite and producing weight loss. Here are a few ways you can optimise your gut microbiome.

More of the good, less of the not-so-good
Increase your intake of healthy whole foods (e.g. fruit, vegetables, wholegrain breads, pastas, and lean meat, chicken and fish) and lower your intake of highly processed and sugary foods (aka 'sometimes foods').

Don't forget the fibre

In perimenopause, aim for at least 25 grams of fibre per day. Fibre is a superfood when it comes to supporting a healthy gut. But it is not just that. Eating foods high in soluble fibre slows digestion and helps you stay fuller for longer. Fibre also supports a healthy functioning liver, which benefits better oestrogen metabolism. Soluble fibre, found in plant foods such as fruits, vegetables, oats, barley and legumes, binds to oestrogen in the gastrointestinal tract and helps clear excess levels from the body via the stools, which can assist with hormone fluctuations. To reach your daily fibre target, focus on eating many of the foods we have discussed in this chapter such as whole grains, beans, lentils, fruits and vegetables.

Include gut-healthy foods every day

It's all about getting prebiotics, probiotics and fermented foods! Probiotics are live microorganisms that have health benefits when consumed in the right amounts (or doses). Certain strains of probiotics have different health benefits. Fermented foods are produced through microbial fermentation. Although not all fermented foods contain probiotics, they still have some gut health benefits. Prebiotic foods have the power to feed the gut microorganisms to keep them happy. In short, the gut is a happier place when there is a good supply of these types of foods.

Probiotic foods: Specific strains and doses of probiotics are added to food sources to provide health benefits – check the label for the word 'probiotic' with the strain listed. Often, probiotics are found added to yoghurt or kefir.

Fermented foods: Tempeh, miso, kimchi, sauerkraut and pickles.

Prebiotic foods: Garlic, onion, leek, shallots, spring onion, chickpeas, lentils, red kidney beans, baked beans, barley, wheat bran, cashews and pistachio nuts.

> **TIP**
>
> A special type of dietary fibre known as resistant starch – that resists digestion in the small intestine – acts as a prebiotic. Foods rich in resistant starch include lentils, beans, peas, whole grains, cooked and cooled potato, rice or pasta and unripe green bananas.

What is the estrobolome?

The estrobolome is a group of gut bacteria that help manage oestrogen in the body. These bacteria make special enzymes that can recycle oestrogen by turning it back into its active form for the body to use again, and they also help break down and remove extra oestrogen to keep hormone levels balanced. This balance between recycling and excreting oestrogen is important for overall health. If your gut bacteria become unbalanced, it can disrupt this process and affect your hormone levels, which may contribute to health problems, especially during perimenopause and menopause, when hormone levels naturally change. Recent large studies show that perimenopause and menopause can change the types of gut bacteria and their ability to process oestrogen, which may be linked to higher risks for heart and metabolic issues in women after menopause. While scientists are still learning about all the ways the estrobolome affects health, keeping your gut healthy may help support balanced hormone levels, particularly during and after menopause.

Tactic 9

CALCIUM PLUS D FOR STRONG BONES

IN A NUTSHELL: Ensure you get your calcium and vitamin D through food and safe sunlight exposure.

HELPS WITH: Reducing the risk, or slowing progression, of osteoporosis.

While this tactic may not make you feel better in the short term, it is one you will thank yourself for later. With lower levels of oestrogen comes reduced calcium absorption which can weaken your bones. While the impacts of weakened bones may not surface until post-menopause (i.e. osteoporosis), the best time to start optimising your diet for strong bones is now. Making sure you have enough calcium and vitamin D is a great way to do this.

Include calcium-rich foods daily

Add serves of dairy to your day. Milk and yoghurt are great options along with cheese in moderation. Or you may choose soy milk which is fortified with calcium as a good option, as you then also get your dose of phytoestrogens. For all plant-based milks, check they are fortified with calcium and shake well before use. Between the ages of 19 and 50, women should aim for 1,000 mg of calcium in the diet daily, and 1,300 mg from 50 and beyond. As an example, a glass of calcium-fortified soy milk or dairy milk usually contains around 200-300 milligrams of calcium. Aim to build up your levels throughout the day with a variety of sources.

Other calcium sources include: Firm tofu, almonds, Brazil nuts, fish with edible bones (such as sardines) and green leafy vegetables.

Don't forget your D

Like a match made in heaven, calcium and vitamin D are the perfect pair. Vitamin D helps your body absorb calcium. This vitamin comes from sunlight, so get some when you can, but don't forget to be sun smart at the same time. Vitamin D is not found in good amounts in many foods. It can be found in fatty fish like sardines and herring, egg yolks and liver. However, a neat trick you may not know is that you can boost the vitamin D content of mushrooms by 'tanning them'. Put your mushrooms in the midday sun for just 15 minutes and this boosts their D. Store in the fridge for up to a week to reap the benefits of your efforts!

—

We've covered a lot of great nutrition tactics in this section. It's OK if you feel overwhelmed at this stage, but I encourage you to let it settle. You won't be adding all nine tactics as part of your Action Plan. Pick and choose, then gradually over time you may find yourself nailing all of them. Take it one step at a time.

Setting yourself up for peri-success

You have the details of what nutrition changes will better support your body in this phase of life. So, what do you need to do to help make some of these changes actually happen? There are some simple things you can do to better propel your success. I've found that one of the simplest ways to make dietary changes is ensuring you have access to the right ingredients in your pantry and fridge so they're all at your fingertips. Having a well-stocked kitchen means you have nourishing products ready when you need a snack or when cooking a quick weeknight meal.

Stock your kitchen

It's time to stock up with perimenopause staples to help power you towards your goals. In this section you'll find my top pantry products to help support your body through this life transition.

TOP TIP

Many clients tell me they have trouble deciphering nutrition panels on food. That's why I created this tool to compare similar products and decide which is best. For example, put two different tomato sauce brands side-by-side, and you can start to see how much sugar some brands add to products like this!

NUTRITION TOOLS AND TACTICS

NUTRITION INFORMATION		
SERVINGS PER PACK: 6	SERVING SIZE: 25 g	
AVG. QUANTITY PER SERVING		PER 100 g
ENERGY	445 kJ (105 Cal)	1780 kJ (425 Cal)
PROTEIN	6.8 g	27.0 g
- gluten	not detected	not detected
FAT - Total	3.9 g	15.7 g
- saturated	0.3 g	1.4 g
CARBOHYDRATE	9.1 g	36.4 g
- sugars	0.5 g	2.2 g
FIBRE	3.8 g	15.0 g
SODIUM	62 mg	250 mg

Check the per 100 g column:

1. Is the sugar <5g/100g?
2. Is the saturated fat <5g/100g?
3. Is the sodium <120mg/100g?

It can sometimes be challenging to find a product that meets all three levels. Aim for products that meet at least two out of three, and where you cannot, compare like-for-like and choose the product that has lower levels of sugar, saturated fat and/or salt.

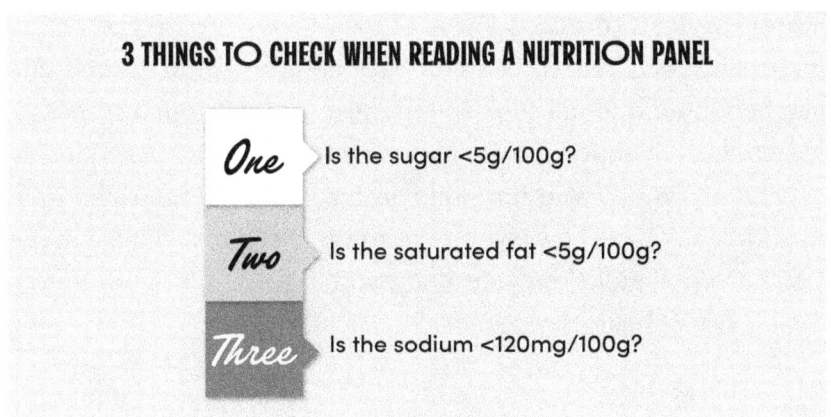

Why are sugar, saturated fat and salt an issue?

Out of the list on a nutrition panel, why have I singled out sugar, saturated fat and salt? Put simply, these three are the things we tend to eat too much of, probably because they make things taste delicious. They are also linked to various health conditions and if reduced in the diet, this can also lower your risk of chronic diseases such as heart disease, stroke, type 2 diabetes, some cancers and chronic kidney disease.

Sugar

Foods and drinks high in sugar are often very energy dense (high in calories), so consuming a lot of them in your diet can make it hard to manage weight. They have also been linked with tooth decay. As you learnt earlier, hormonal changes in perimenopause may cause insulin resistance. This makes it harder for your body to move sugar from the blood into the cells so it can be utilised. Over time, insulin resistance may lead to a diagnosis of type 2 diabetes.

Saturated fat

Eating too much saturated fat (fats that are solid at room temperature) can lead to raised levels of bad cholesterol in the blood, increasing your risk of heart disease and stroke. Saturated fats can be found in foods such as red meat, chicken, butter, cheese, ice-cream, coconut oil, palm oil, and some fried and baked foods. As you now know, your hormone oestrogen levels drop over time in perimenopause. Low levels of oestrogen lead to a change in the way fats are handled by your body, and in turn, this is linked to a higher risk of heart disease.

Salt

Too much salt in your diet can cause water retention and increase blood pressure. Aim to eat no more than one teaspoon of salt per day, which is equivalent to 2,000 milligrams of sodium. It really is such a small amount. That's why it is a good idea to keep an eye on added salt in packaged foods. The risk of heart disease and high blood pressure increases during menopause. That, along with research showing that menopausal women become more sensitive to the impacts of salt on blood pressure, means it is even more important to be aware of how much salt you are consuming daily.

TIP

Choose products that contain less than 120 mg of sodium per 100 grams. On a nutrition panel, salt is listed as sodium. While the terms are often used interchangeably, they are not the same. The chemical name for salt is sodium chloride – it contains about 40% sodium and 60% chloride. The sodium component of salt is linked with negative health effects, which is why it is listed on the label.

Action Step
PERIMENOPAUSE PANTRY STAPLES

Look through your pantry and see what you're missing. Next time you go shopping, add in some peri-beneficial staples. You can do this over a few weeks to reduce the burden on your hip pocket.

FRUIT AND VEGGIES

- Canned or tinned veggies with low added salt and no added sugar, e.g. edamame, four bean mix, chickpeas, black beans, lentils
- Dried legumes and soak before use
- Canned or dried fruits with no added sugar

BREADS, GRAINS AND CEREALS

Smart carb options:

- Wholegrain breads, wraps, crisps or thins
- Soy-linseed bread or crackers
- Pumpernickel bread
- Wheat, rice or oat bran to make porridges
- Protein rich pasta, e.g. pulse pasta
- Low carb noodles, e.g. edamame bean spaghetti
- Whole grain or brown basmati rice, low GI rice, wild rice
- Quinoa
- Soba noodles
- Mung bean noodles
- Freekah
- Barley

NUTRITION TOOLS AND TACTICS

- Bulgur (cracked wheat)
- Chickpea flour
- Traditional rolled or steel-cut oats, e.g. for homemade muesli, muesli bars or porridge
  Keep on hand a mixture of nuts and seeds (low or no added salt varieties) to make your own muesli or granola. See my Instagram for a perimenopause powered muesli recipe.

SNACK FOODS

- Muesli bars or snack/protein bars that are nut based (tend to be lower in added sugar)
- Unsalted and unflavoured nuts and seeds, e.g. pistachios, cashews, almonds, hazelnuts, walnuts, chia seeds, hemp seeds, sunflower seeds and flaxseeds (aka linseeds)
  Pistachios are a good source of melatonin – the sleep-regulating hormone. Try a handful before bed.
- Unhulled sesame seeds (these are higher in calcium than the hulled variety)
- Wholegrain thins or crisps (soy-linseed is a great option)

FLAVOURED DRINKS

- Sparkling water/low or no sugar drinks
- Black coffee, decaffeinated coffee, caffeine free herbal teas, e.g. iced tea with a flavour like green apple or pomegranate

SAUCES, SPREADS, COOKING OILS AND OTHER CONDIMENTS

- Varieties of vinegar to create healthy salad dressings
  And despite what you may see on social media, you don't need to drink apple cider vinegar every day to keep your blood sugar in check.

- Natural nut butters made from 100 percent nuts with a little added salt as the only other ingredient
    Note that saturated fat levels may be higher than 5g/100g as nuts are naturally high in fats. Avoid any products that contain added sugar.
- Extra virgin olive oil – see more on this later

Great seasoning options are:
- Seaweed flakes
- Nutritional yeast
- Reduced salt soy sauce
- Herbs and spices – especially turmeric and cinnamon

CHOCOLATE, DESSERTS AND SWEET TREATS

Options that satisfy a sweet craving, and also power you in perimenopause:
- Low or no added sugar dried fruits, nut bars or other muesli bars
- Cacao powder
    Simply add a few teaspoons of cacao, some honey or monk fruit sweetener, your warmed milk of choice, and make a nourishing hot chocolate (that's packed with powerful antioxidants for an added health boost).

NUTRITION TOOLS AND TACTICS

Ingredient spotlight on extra virgin olive oil

When it comes to pantry staples, you cannot go past extra virgin olive oil (EVOO). It's versatile, healthy and most importantly delicious. Before you ask ... yes, you can cook with it. Good quality, local, fresh EVOO is tolerant to heat and can be used to fry, bake, grill and barbeque. It is most delicious when served fresh as part of a salad dressing, or as a topper to pasta, avocado on toast or whatever you please. Research shows that daily use of one to two tablespoons of EVOO has enormous heart health benefits, important in perimenopause. In addition, diets high in EVOO (as part of a Mediterranean diet pattern) can help reduce the severity and intensity of hot flushes while providing brain-boosting benefits to help combat emotional stress, anxiety and brain fog. Do you need any more reasons to include this in your diet every day? While you may think you need other oils in your pantry, EVOO can pretty much do it all. One caveat is that you choose a high quality, local EVOO to reap the full benefits.

Here is a quick checklist:

- ☐ Choose an oil that is locally produced with fresh grown olives, e.g. your local state, neighbourhood or suburb, if you are so lucky!

- ☐ Look for a best-before date on the label. Some cooking oils do not include these! But, being a fat source, these break down and become rancid (i.e. they go bad).

- ☐ Avoid any product that has no best-before or expiry date and opt for a brand that also prints a harvest date, so you know when the olives were picked from the tree. After all, the olive is a fruit, right? So, like all other fruits, once it's picked from the tree, it starts to lose its goodness. You want olives that are picked and pressed to EVOO as fast as humanly possible.

In terms of other oils

Watch out for oils labelled only olive oil, or blended olive oil. These are not as natural as EVOO and do undergo processing which strips some of the natural antioxidants.

Vegetable and seed oils: Canola oil, rapeseed oil and rice bran oil are heavily processed. These oils are produced with chemicals to help extract the oil from the plants used. Although not 100 percent proven by research, there is some concern these oils also promote inflammation and poor health outcomes in the body.

Coconut oil: Solid at room temperature, this oil mainly contains saturated fat and is not overly rich in antioxidants. If you use coconut oil as a base for protein balls, as it is solid at room temperature, simply swap for EVOO and store them in the fridge!

Eat like a Mediterranean

Solid research shows the Mediterranean diet has a positive effect on many areas of health, including heart and brain health, which is good news in perimenopause. How can you be more Med? Place a greater emphasis on plant-based foods and healthy fats (cue EVOO!). The Mediterraneans pack their plates with veggies, fruits and whole grains, eat a good amount of omega-3 rich fish (e.g. tuna, salmon and mackerel), a moderate amount of cheese and yoghurt and little or no red meat. Their protein of choice is usually beans, fish or poultry. As you can see, it is very peri-friendly! Along with this, the diet has few sweets, sugary drinks or butter and, of course, has a moderate amount of wine, consumed with meals. This dietary pattern also contains many healthy ingredients like

NUTRITION TOOLS AND TACTICS

EVOO, tomato, herbs and spices, garlic and onions, which contain natural bio-active substances to help reduce inflammation and protect from free radicals that can damage body cells, leading to poor health.

Action Step
FRIDGE AND FREEZER STAPLES

Time to check your cooler. What can you add to your next grocery shop to boost the peri-goodness, while enjoying nourishing and versatile ingredients?

YOGHURT AND OTHER CREAMY OPTIONS

- Natural or Greek yoghurts, high protein yoghurts and/or high protein puddings with low levels of added sugar
- Kefir
  Look for yoghurts and kefir with added probiotic strains for extra gut health and other benefits.
- Cottage cheese
  This is packed with protein and lower in calories than most other cheeses. It's also a versatile ingredient that can be used as a spread, dip, in baked dishes and more. However, it can be high in salt.

MILK

- Dairy and soy milk have high levels of protein per serve
- If choosing plant-based milk alternatives, look for ones with little to no additives, and products fortified with calcium for bone health
  Consider trying soy milk as this also contains phytoestrogens.

SPREADS, CONDIMENTS AND SAUCES

- Unsalted butter – to be used in moderation
  When it comes to spreadable butters, look for products that only contain cream and maybe some salt. Triple-churned cream and salt = spreadable butter, no additives needed!
- Try substituting butter or other spreads with dips like hummus, cream cheese or avocado

- Miso, kimchi, sauerkraut and pickles
- Full-fat mayonnaise with minimal additives – enjoy in moderation
- Sauces lower in salt and sugar, or no added sugar options where possible

FRUITS AND VEGGIES

- Snap-frozen vegetables
  Often higher in nutrients as they are usually picked at peak ripeness and frozen soon after, they are great options for a quick stir fry, to bulk out soups and curries and for many other creations.
- Cauliflower and/or broccoli rice are great freezer options to bulk out or replace rice
- Frozen edamame is a great option to have on hand for salads, stir fries or snacks
- Low GI fruits and veggies, e.g. sweet potato, capsicum, broccoli, asparagus, mushrooms, zucchini, spinach, cauliflower, green beans, lettuce, cucumbers, celery, tomato, onion, eggplant, cabbage, sweet corn, parsnips, taro, apples, oranges, grapes, apricots, plums, kiwis, peaches, pears and nectarines
- Prebiotic options: garlic, onion, leek, shallots, spring onion

PROTEINS TO BUILD MEALS AROUND

- Fresh free-range eggs – a great protein source with versatility for meals and snacks
- Other protein sources such as lean chicken, meat, fish, tofu, tempeh
  Tofu and tempeh also contain phytoestrogens.

SWEET TREATS

- Lower added-sugar ice creams and frozen desserts – enjoy in moderation
- High-protein yoghurt as an ice-cream swap
  Add the yoghurt to moulds, pop in a stick and freeze, add fresh cut fruit and honey for extra sweetness, or use flavoured low sugar yoghurt varieties.

How does it all come together?

One step at a time. Change is incremental, and it is unrealistic to think you can add all nine tactics to your diet and revamp your pantry, fridge and freezer immediately. All these tactics and tips are your ultimate guide to managing the symptoms of perimenopause. Remember, you will choose tactics to match up with your SMART goals in Chapter 6 and focus on them for the next 3-6 months. This is a cyclical process. You will be back reviewing nutritional tactics when you repeat the steps and move towards new goals in later stages of perimenopause.

What I can promise is that this process is self-fulfilling. Our bodily systems are intertwined and all impact each other. Even implementing one or two tactics will lead to change, and from that you can feel motivated to add a few more tactics and reap the benefits. You may have noticed a trend in this chapter. The focus is on what you *can* include in your diet, how you *can enjoy* all types of foods, and not what you need to avoid or restrict. There are some foods and drinks you may wish to limit, and some you may wilfully choose to eliminate as you notice how they impact your symptoms. But you do not have to cut out food groups unless there is a medical reason to do so. Crowd your plate with delicious, nourishing and hormone-balancing foods and you will help ease symptoms of brain fog, low energy, mood changes, hot flushes, night sweats and more. Nutrition is the foundation of your cake.

From here, we'll look at lifestyle changes, the role of HRT and supplements.

SUMMARY OF NUTRITION TOOLS AND TACTICS

SUMMARY OF TACTIC	HELPS WITH	RELEVANT TO MY GOALS Y/N
Hit your protein targets, spread evenly throughout the day. 1-1.2 grams of protein per kilo of body weight per day.	Weight control, muscle growth and maintenance, blood sugar control.	
Pack your plate with smart carbs to help slow digestion, providing sustained energy.	Weight control, blood sugar control, low energy levels.	
Eat as many different plant foods as possible.	Weight control, blood sugar control, low energy levels, brain fog, heart health, gut health.	
Add in 1-2 servings of phytoestrogen rich foods each day to support hormone balance.	Hormonal symptoms (i.e. mood changes, brain fog, hot flushes).	
Include omega-3 rich food in your diet for brain health and a healthy heart.	Brain fog, mood changes, heart and cholesterol health.	
Choose foods rich in B vitamins and iron to help elevate your energy levels.	Brain fog, low energy levels.	

SUMMARY OF TACTIC	HELPS WITH	RELEVANT TO MY GOALS Y/N
Aim for at least 8-10 glasses of water a day, while limiting alcohol and caffeine.	Weight control, brain fog, mood changes, low energy levels.	
Nourish your gut health with whole foods, fermented foods, prebiotics and probiotics.	Weight control, low energy levels, mood changes, brain fog.	
Love your bones with calcium and vitamin D.	Stronger bones to help prevent osteoporosis.	

Clinical case: Emma's evolution

All case studies are based on real client experiences. Names and personal details have been changed for privacy.

Emma, aged 41, has been following fad diets all her life. From weight watchers as a younger adult, to the soup diet, intermittent fasting and keto, she has tried them all. At 68 kg, Emma is a healthy weight, but feels she constantly struggles to keep her weight stable, so restricts foods, and beats herself up when she has too many sweet treats. She came to me to learn more about intuitive eating, as she had noticed in the past year that midline belly fat had started to increase and her PMS was off the charts. She wanted to feel free when eating food and not worried all the time, while better regulating her mood at that time of the month.

Emma's story was not unfamiliar. Many women who grew up in the 90s were sold low-fat diets as the key to looking good at all costs. Emma worked with me for over two years and together we discovered she was under-fuelling most days, fasting on days after a big meal due to guilt, eating lots of low-calorie/low-fat foods that were usually high in additives and low in essential nutrients, and avoiding carbs, even though she absolutely loved bread and pasta, being of Italian descent. Together, we wiped the slate clean of all the diet noise and influence she had heard over the years and focused on her two goals: eating in a less restrictive way and managing her PMS. The most successful tactics were levelling up protein (especially at breakfast), adding in smart carbs (including bread and pasta) for enjoyment and nourishment and adding in phytoestrogens. I recently asked Emma how she felt now that we had implemented these tactics over a longer period, and here is what she said.

Emma: I have gone from worrying about every food choice I make to feeling a sense of freedom. I think about what I can eat and what I should eat to help my body thrive, versus what I need to avoid and eliminate. Overall, being kinder to myself is a much nicer way to be than how I was before. I love that pasta, bread and sweet foods are all still part of my day. It's just about balance and choosing foods that power me well. I love packing protein into my day in creative ways, as I feel satisfied, and my muscle definition is improving as well. My belly fat has reduced and my old jeans fit. I don't even weigh myself now. If my clothes fit, I am happy, as I was too hard on myself before when I fluctuated in weight. And as for the PMS, if I miss adding in my flaxseeds and eating tofu, etc. especially when travelling for work, I notice a massive change in my mood fluctuations, so I think it's working for me!

Chapter 4
LIFESTYLE SHIFTS THAT MAKE A DIFFERENCE

• • • • • • • • • • • • •

SOPHIA tucks into bed and reflects on the day. She ate well today, and it felt good to have more energy. But there are a few things weighing on her mind this evening. She's in a constant state of worry, more so than usual. Her parent's deteriorating health is weighing on her and sometimes she gets ravelled in thoughts and feels her chest tighten. Then there's the ever-growing to-do list that triggers her anxious mind. There are not enough hours in the day. She used to take it all in her stride, but nowadays she's more easily overwhelmed. It would be nice to try to relax a little more. Her sister told her about a special breathing technique that calms the body. *Maybe that is worth a try?* And then there's the whole waking at 3 am every night thing. Like clockwork, Sophia can guarantee she'll be wide awake and scrolling social media in the early hours of the morning. Sometimes she can fall back asleep, but other times she just scrolls away until it's time to get up. It's definitely racing thoughts that stop her from getting back to sleep again. She makes a mental note to ask the doctor if there is anything else she can do for all of this? Last week, Sophia heard a great podcast that talked about the benefits of exercise for sleep.

Not really sure how exercise and sleep are related? One to explore when she gets a moment.

Sophia wonders, *when did it all become so different?* Looking back, life in her early-30s was a lot simpler. None of this perimenopause stuff to deal with. Every now and then she might have a bit of anxiety and a few sleepless nights. Now, it seems that the simplest things are a lot harder to manage. It feels like her body needs a little extra help to get through things these days. But, Sophia is hopeful. She knows she can use science-based tactics to help her body through this life stage.

• • • • • • • • • • • • •

Like Sophia, you will be experiencing your own unique set of perimenopause symptoms. Many women tell me that heightened anxiety and stress, mood changes and disturbed sleep are some of the most troublesome symptoms. While you can strengthen the foundations of your cake (aka the flour), you need to work out how to bind the flour together, forming a nice, smooth batter. Time for the eggs, butter and milk – your lifestyle tactics. These are what help bolster your revised nutrition tactics to manage symptoms.

What exactly are 'lifestyle tactics'? These are your daily habits and routines that play a critical role in overall health, including areas such as sleep patterns, physical activity and stress management. Unpacking each of these lifestyle areas can expose habits you have developed over time, which may not be serving you well right now. Adding in tactics across self-care, sleep, stress management and movement have all been shown to improve symptoms. Depending on your SMART goals, each of these tactics will have a varying level of importance when it comes to the ones you adopt. Take this next section as a good opportunity to reflect on these areas of your life and decide if any of these lifestyle changes could boost your wellbeing. As a reminder, in Chapter 6, we will match your selected tactics across nutrition and lifestyle to your goals to create an Action Plan.

The mental load

Let's take a moment to discuss mental health and the emotional toll that perimenopause can take on your life. For some, it can be described as an identity crisis. You just don't feel like your old self. While some tactics in this chapter are designed to soothe your nervous system and help with the emotions that come with this major life change, I highly recommend you seek support from a psychologist if you need it. I can assure you that it's not all in your head. You likely feel different, things seem a little harder to manage at times, and you are experiencing lots of different and new symptoms and emotions.

5 top lifestyle tactics
FOR PERIMENOPAUSE

Tactic 1

SELF-CARE, MEDITATION AND MINDFULNESS

TACTIC IN A NUTSHELL: Add some meditation and mindfulness to your day to reap the benefits.

HELPS WITH: Mood changes, increased stress, sleep disturbances, hot flushes, night sweats, aches and pains.

Self-care and mindfulness are just two tactics that may help support you when it comes to mental wellbeing. What exactly is self-care? It's best described as conscious acts that one takes to promote physical, mental, spiritual and emotional health. Acts of self-care ensure a strong mind-body connection and can have a powerful impact on health. When it comes to perimenopause, two self-care practices that have specific benefits are meditation and mindfulness. Mindfulness is simply a form of meditation that helps you focus on being aware of your thoughts, sensations and surroundings in the moment, without interpretation or judgment. Meditation and mindfulness can be helpful in promoting relaxation, as well as soothing symptoms such as hot flushes, night sweats, mood changes, sleep disturbances, aches and pains. What's more is that meditation and mindfulness have been shown to lower cortisol (the stress hormone) to exert their relaxing effect, somewhat combating rising levels that occur in midlife. Here are some easy ways to include self-care tactics in your day.

LIFESTYLE SHIFTS THAT MAKE A DIFFERENCE

Find a meditation podcast and try to stick to it as a daily habit or routine. My favourites are *Mindful in Minutes*, *Calm* and *Headspace*.

Invest in activities such as colouring or painting to help keep you in the moment and have more time away from screens.

Try deep breathing exercises when feeling stressed or anxious. Here is one simple breathing technique. Box breathing helps to relax your mind and calm your nervous system. It helps to visualise four sides of a box when you try this.

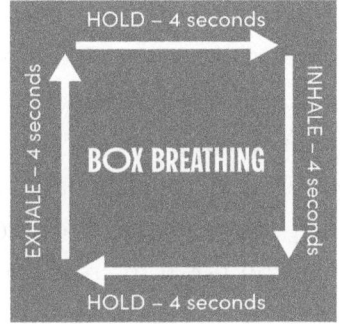

Breathe in while counting to four and notice the air filling your lungs.

Hold your breath for four seconds.

Slowly exhale through your mouth while counting to four.

Pause your breath for four seconds.

Repeat these four steps until you feel more relaxed and centred.

Why stress management is so important in perimenopause

The hypothalamic-pituitary-adrenal axis, or HPA axis, is a communication system in the body that controls the response to stress. A reduction in progesterone during perimenopause is thought to destabilise this stress response system. Lifestyle changes will play a role in helping the body cope with this change and support your stress response and overall wellbeing.

Tactic 2

ESTABLISH A SLEEP ROUTINE

TACTIC IN A NUTSHELL: Nail your sleep routine and be conscious of sleep detractors that could be impacting your rest.

HELPS WITH: Sleep disturbances, low energy levels, brain fog.

Your sleep depends on what is called the circadian rhythm, a 24-hour sleep-wake cycle which acts as your body's internal clock. Hormones play a role here again, mainly melatonin and cortisol, when it comes to sleep. Not getting enough sleep can impact many other areas of your health such as reducing energy levels and causing brain fog. Lifestyle tactics for better sleep help nurture your circadian rhythm, supporting you more easily to wind down for rest and enjoy a peaceful night's sleep. Sleep hygiene is a term used to describe good sleep habits that help you get some quality rest. This includes your daily routine when it comes to sleep, your environment and other factors that can impact sleep quality, such as timing of meals and use of digital devices. Consider these lifestyle tips for better sleep.

Stick to a sleep schedule
Support your natural sleep-wake cycle by allowing for 7-9 hours of sleep each night. Choose a time to go to bed and wake, and for the most part keep that consistent across your week. While doing this, if you lie in bed and cannot fall asleep within 20 minutes, leave your bedroom and do something relaxing (e.g. meditation or a warm bath) and head back to the bed when you feel more sleepy. Your bed is for sleeping, so try not to read, watch TV or listen to

a podcast in bed. You are best to leave the room and come back, reserving the bed for sleep.

Be aware of the impacts of food, drinks and exercise on sleep

Making sure you don't go to bed feeling too hungry or too full can help you avoid unnecessary discomfort. Avoid any caffeine or alcohol within 4 hours of bedtime as they can reduce your sleep quality by raising levels of cortisol. While regular physical activity can promote better sleep, avoid vigorous exercises close to bedtime, as this may interfere with winding down and falling asleep.

Create a restful environment

Your room should be dark, cool and quiet to optimise sleep. If you are experiencing night sweats or hot flushes, make sure you have lighter blankets or sheets, and choose light, loose and breathable fabrics for your sleepwear. Natural fibres such as wool or linen are good choices. Having access to a fan or cooling may also help if you find yourself in a pool of sweat at 3 am.

Unplug before bed

Close or switch off any digital devices or screens (i.e. TV, phones, tablets, laptops) at least one hour before your scheduled sleep time. Your natural melatonin levels rise around two hours prior to bedtime. Continuing to look at screens right up until you try to sleep exposes you to blue and green light that can neutralise the sleepy effects of melatonin, affecting your sleep quality. That also means you should stop reaching for your phone if you wake during the night. This may be easier said than done. Think of ways to make it easier, e.g. can you leave your phone charging in another room?

Feast your eyes on morning sunlight for better sleep!
Your alarm clock pings at 6 am and you think about reaching straight for your phone to start scrolling. If you're lucky enough to wake when it's daylight, why not leave the phone, open the blinds or step outside and let your eyes take in a dose of the sun and sky for a few blissful moments. If you wake when it's dark, can you prioritise a dose of sunlight when you see it emerge for the day? Research shows that people who get a good dose of natural bright light during the day fall asleep faster and get better quality sleep. In particular, morning sunlight has been shown to help regulate your circadian rhythm to naturally support your sleep-wake cycle.

Tactic 3
REGULAR EXERCISE

TACTIC IN A NUTSHELL: Each week, schedule a balanced amount of strength training with cardio, gentle movement and mobility exercises.

HELPS WITH: Muscle and bone health, heart health, low energy levels, sleep disturbances, mood changes, weight control, hormonal symptoms.

Prioritising regular exercise can have a wide range of benefits in midlife. These include boosting energy levels, helping with sleep, reducing heart health risks, maintaining liver health, alleviating stress, supporting a healthy weight, improving hormone-related symptoms, and preserving muscle mass and bone strength. There are so many reasons to prioritise exercise, but the key is finding the right balance for this stage of life. It might be a good idea to work with a qualified exercise professional (e.g. personal trainer or exercise physiologist) to create your plan. But in the meantime, here's a guide:

Include strength (resistance) training at least 2-3 times a week
The drop in oestrogen levels in your body reduces bone strength and muscle mass. Strength training can help build muscle but also helps keep your bones strong. These types of exercises use weights or your own bodyweight to build strength in bones and muscles, like push-ups, squats, lunges, lifting weights or using resistance bands. Keep in mind it doesn't necessarily mean extremely heavy weights for everyone – you really need a personalised plan. This is best done with an exercise professional who can also ensure you have good form and technique, helping avoid unnecessary injuries. Even better is if you can find someone who is experienced in women's health and training.

Daily movement for the win
If chasing that 10,000 step goal motivates you, then keep at it, but it may be easier to deliberately increase incidental movement to up your step count. Choosing to walk around the block in your lunch break, getting off at an earlier train station, or walking around the house while chatting on the phone are all ways to get moving. You may even like to invest in a walking pad to get some extra steps in while you're at home. This gentle, low-pace movement is good for your body but also keeps your mind clear and supports mental clarity.

Balance it all out
For those of us who grew up in the 90s, aerobic cardio workouts were all the rage. While these have a place, it is a good idea not to flood your week with high-intensity training, as this can overstress your body and lead to fatigue. Short bursts of cardio (e.g. a

20-minute jog or a 30-minute high-intensity class) can be good for your heart health and more, but in this phase of life, try not to overdo it and keep a good balance. My biggest tip here is to find something you love. Jogging, running, dance classes, tennis, basketball – the list goes on. If you don't love it, you won't stick with it to make a regular healthy habit.

Also be sure to save and dedicate some time to rest and recovery. Why not try an infrared sauna, spa, yoga or breathwork class? A weekly plan might look like this:

- 2–3 strength sessions (e.g. 30–45 minutes using weights under the guidance of an exercise professional)
- 1–3 short cardio sessions a week (e.g. 20–30 minutes of running, power walking, gym class, tennis etc.)
- Daily walking of 20–30 minutes (minimum)
- Optional mobility work, e.g. Pilates, stretching
- Don't forget to schedule in time for rest and recovery too

Benefits of a weighted vest for walking

You may have heard of weighted vests. What are they, and do they benefit women in perimenopause? These wearable vests usually offer between 5 and 10 kg of extra weight that can be easily worn during exercise. These vests have a multitude of benefits for women as we age. Although most research in this space is in post-menopausal women, there's no reason why you cannot try a weighted vest in perimenopause to reap benefits such as increased lower-body muscle strength and power, and lower risk of falls later in life. As reduced bone strength typically comes with menopause, bone breaks and fractures can cause significant health and mobility issues. Longer-term exercise using weighted vests (5 years plus) in post-menopausal women is associated with less bone loss, meaning bones remain stronger with age. Weighted vests can play a role in boosting muscle strength whilst reaping the other benefits of low intensity and incidental exercise, such as walking or gardening. A good goal is to gradually increase the weight in your vest until you reach around 5-10 percent of your body weight. Take care to adjust slowly, and take regular breaks when walking, especially as you get used to the additional load. If you ramp up the weight too fast, or go too hard, you risk injury. Slow and steady does it.

TIP

Did you know that time in nature may benefit your nervous system? Why not walk, meditate or read a book outside amongst the greenery or other natural spaces. This has been shown to reduce stress, have a calming effect and improve your overall mood.

Tactic 4
LIMIT ENDOCRINE-DISRUPTING CHEMICALS

TACTIC IN A NUTSHELL: Choose cosmetics and household products that are free from phthalates and parabens.

HELPS WITH: Hormonal fluctuations.

Can your makeup, skincare, cookware and other household products impact hormones? Lifestyle tips to support hormone balance can come in many shapes and forms. This one may seem a bit off centre, but stick with me. Before I start, please don't madly rush around the house and throw away products that contain the discussed ingredients or go down a Google rabbit warren on how to 'cleanse' or 'rid' your house of toxins. Quite frankly, this topic could be a book on its own. What's good to know is that there are some ingredients, perfumes, plastics and other substances that have 'endocrine-disrupting' properties. This means they could potentially disrupt your hormone balance, and in perimenopause, they may contribute to the overall decline in oestrogen over time.

A good place to start is looking for any products you have (beauty, skincare, household cleaners and the like) that contain phthalates or parabens. You ideally want to avoid or limit any products that contain these. Try to replace products as they run out with more natural products that are free from endocrine-disrupting ingredients as you go. Your hormones will thank you for it! Perhaps start with your cosmetic and skincare products. Anything you apply to your skin can absorb into the bloodstream.

What are parabens and phthalates?
Parabens are often used as preservatives to extend shelf life in personal care products. It is thought that they can mimic oestrogen by potentially binding to oestrogen receptors.

Phthalates are chemicals that help increase the flexibility and durability of plastics. They are commonly found in self-care products (e.g. shampoo and soap), fragrances and plastics. Phthalates can have adverse effects on reproductive tissues in the body and are believed to play a role in reducing oestrogen and testosterone levels.

How to check for phthalates and parabens
Choose products that have labelling, such as phthalate-free or 0% phthalates, paraben-free or 0% parabens. The most common

parabens found in cosmetics are methylparaben, propylparaben, butylparaben and ethylparaben. Check the ingredient list. The following examples are what you will see if a product contains phthalates:

- DINP (diisononyl phthalate)
- DEP (diethyl phthalate)
- DEHP (di-2-ethylhexyl phthalate)
- DMP (dimethyl phthalate)
- BBP (benzyl butyl phthalate)
- DNOP (di-n-octyl phthalate)
- DIDP (diisodecyl phthalate)

If in doubt, contact the manufacturer and ask if the product contains any phthalates or parabens.

Ever heard of xenoestrogens?
Xenoestrogens are natural or synthetic chemicals that mimic oestrogen in the body and have the potential to impact hormone balance. Xenoestrogens can be found in a variety of products such as pesticides, plastics, and personal care and household products. Phthalates and parabens are considered xenoestrogens, as well as bisphenol A (BPA), which is found in containers that store food and beverages, such as water bottles, and also commonly coats the inside of food cans, bottle tops and more.

In reality, it is almost impossible to avoid all endocrine-disrupting chemicals. However, in addition to being more aware of phthalates, parabens and other xenoestrogens, here are a few ways to limit your exposure:

- Limit your consumption of food and beverages packed in plastic.

- Try not to keep canned or plastic-wrapped foods in hot areas (e.g. the car) and avoid reheating food in plastic containers.
- Find BPA-free products.
- Choose fragrance-free products or opt for products that use pure essential oils.
- Wash fruit and vegetables with water and/or a low-tox cleaning product before consuming. Even better, choose organic fruits and vegetables that are less likely to be treated with synthetic pesticides or herbicides. If you grow your own veggies, only use natural pesticide products.
- If possible, use filtered tap water.

Tactic 5

MEDICAL TREATMENTS

TACTIC IN A NUTSHELL: Speak to your trusted doctor to see if HRT or other treatments are suitable for you.

HELPS WITH: Many symptoms across the board.

As we round out this section on lifestyle tactics, it would be remiss of me not to mention medical treatments, the potential icing to your cake!

What about HRT or the pill?

A key part of your health and lifestyle routine should be regular contact with a general practitioner (GP). They help bring all facets of your health together, see the big picture and work with you

LIFESTYLE SHIFTS THAT MAKE A DIFFERENCE

on your overall health and wellbeing. Medical treatments can be one of the most effective ways to manage the symptoms of perimenopause. However, there are many nuances and schools of thought when it comes to the use of HRT, and even the oral contraceptive pill (the pill), to provide symptom relief. The information in this section is designed to arm you with the right amount of knowledge, so you can start a conversation with your GP about perimenopause.

TIP

Find the right doctor for you! Do your research and find out if your GP has a special interest in women's health and perimenopause or menopause. If not, can they recommend someone else to help you on this journey?

What do you need to know about HRT and the pill?

HRT and the pill are treatment options for perimenopause that you can get from your doctor. Over the past few decades, there has been much debate about how safe HRT is and which type best helps manage symptoms. The information below is designed to help you have a conversation with your doctor about this, and provides a summary of pros, cons and the history when it comes to medications.

In 2002, a very large study called the Women's Health Initiative (WHI) was abruptly stopped after 5.6 years. The way this study's findings were shared by the media had a dramatic effect on the use of HRT, and this still lingers to this day. Let's unpack some of the key facts here.

This study was designed to discover if older women (average age of 63 years) who started on HRT would receive the same heart health benefits as younger women. The results showed a relatively small increased risk of breast cancer when older (more synthetic) forms of HRT were used (more on that soon). Long story short, the media took these results and created headlines claiming that HRT significantly increased the risk of breast cancer, among other things, in post-menopausal women. At the same time, they completely downplayed the positive effects, like reduced risk of fractures and colorectal cancer.

In fact, when the data was looked at later, women aged between 50 and 59 experienced many benefits of HRT and had fewer cancers and fractures than women taking the placebo. Also keep in mind that when it comes to perimenopause, women are typically much younger than the average age in the WHI study and are generally the ones experiencing highly troublesome symptoms. Essentially, it is important to bear in mind that the study itself was not designed to look at the safety or efficacy of HRT use in perimenopause – it was mainly to determine heart health benefits for older women.

However, the related media storm left a mess in its wake. Women of all ages and stages of menopause threw away their HRT and were fearful of it. Doctors were also left scared to prescribe it and this lingers in the way some doctors, as well as women, think about HRT today.

There is now more research and newer forms of HRT, and on the whole, the benefits usually outweigh the risks. Many women in perimenopause feel much better on HRT whilst also enjoying the protective benefits it has for some conditions such as osteoporosis, cardiovascular disease and declines in brain function later in life. It's worth a discussion with your doctor. HRT has some real benefits if started in perimenopause versus waiting until you have endured symptoms for many years with minimal relief.

HRT is not for everyone though, and your doctor will assess your specific case. It may not be suitable if you have had:

- Breast cancer, endometrial cancer or other cancers that are hormone dependent (note: if you have a family history of cancer, your doctor will assess the risk with each treatment option)
- Vaginal bleeding that has not been properly diagnosed
- Blood clots
- Heart disease or stroke
- Liver disease
- High blood pressure that is not treated
- Other conditions as assessed by your doctor

HRT

Let's start with the benefits of HRT. While you certainly don't need to be an expert, knowing a little more about what HRT contains, the formats and a few safety tips can be helpful. Nowadays, most HRT products contain body-identical (also known as bio-identical) forms of oestrogen, in the form of oestradiol. Some products also contain a type of progesterone, either as a synthetic progestin or a body-identical micronised progesterone. Hormones are usually included in HRT at relatively low doses. They are intended to replace what the body is naturally losing and support better hormone balance.

Body-identical means hormones that are the same molecular shape as those produced by the body. They are produced in a laboratory from wild yams, cactus and soy. This is compared to earlier years, when hormones were derived from the urine of pregnant horses! This ingredient reads as 'equine oestrogens' and is still available in Australia at the time of writing this book. The science is still emerging, but it does seem that body-identical hormones have a more favourable safety profile.

HRT comes in a variety of formats. Pills, patches, gels and creams are the main types.

In Australia, regimens for HRT include:

- **Oestrogen only:** For women who have had a hysterectomy. Progesterone has no real benefit for women without a uterus, as its main purpose is to stop the uterine lining from growing out of control.
- **Combined oestrogen plus progestogen:** For women with an intact uterus:
  - **Cyclical continuous oestrogen** with a progestogen given cyclically (e.g. 12 to 14 continuous days of a month).
  - **Continuous combined HRT** of continuous oestrogen and progestogen.

Terminology check

When it comes to HRT, ingredient names can be confusing, especially when referring to hormones that act to replace natural progesterone. Here's a quick breakdown.

Progestins are the name for synthetic versions of progestogen. (Progestogen is the name for a molecule that has some similar effects to progesterone in the body.) Common ingredient names for progestins include levonorgestrel, drospirenone and norethisterone. Although progestins have similar effects as progesterone, they do have other effects that can often be responsible for side effects such as fluid retention, headache and mood disturbances.

Natural progesterone is derived from soybeans, Mexican yam roots, and sometimes from animal ovaries. When included in HRT, this ingredient is called oral micronised progesterone, a format that is better absorbed by the body. It is body-identical, generally well tolerated and not shown to impact mood.

In some cases, women are also prescribed **testosterone** therapy, which is typically added to an HRT regime for low libido.

Additional possible benefits of testosterone therapy include improvements in mood, sleep, muscle mass, concentration and energy levels. Like most hormone therapies, results vary from person to person, with some women reaping no benefits, while others say testosterone is life-changing. Discuss your unique circumstances with your doctor. Unlike most other countries, in Australia there is a specific body-identical testosterone cream available for women. In other locations, women are forced to use formulations designed for men, which come in much higher doses, making it hard to find the right dose for perimenopause or postmenopausal symptoms.

TIP

In Australia, there are many different forms and types of HRT. The Australasian Menopause Society provides a good, up-to-date summary on their website.

In short, the following formats are currently available:

SYSTEMIC HRT: This usually contains higher doses of oestrogen and comes in a variety of formats, including tablets, capsules, transdermal skin patches, gels or vaginal rings. Being systemic means the medicine in these products travels to all parts of your body via the bloodstream. Given its wide-reaching effect, systemic HRT can be helpful for many perimenopause symptoms.

TOPICAL HRT: These varieties usually contain lower-doses of oestrogen. They are available in a range of forms such as creams, pessaries and intrauterine systems that are for the vaginal area. As they are more topical in nature, they are not as easily absorbed throughout the body and mainly have their action in the local tissue. Topical HRT can be specifically helpful for local symptoms such as vaginal dryness.

Side effects

As HRT contains lower doses of hormones, side effects are usually minimal, varying between types and forms, but can include headache, breast pain or tenderness, unexpected vaginal bleeding or spotting, nausea, mood changes including low mood or depression, leg cramps, mild rashes or itching, diarrhoea and hair loss. Many women get effective symptom relief within days to weeks after taking HRT. Starting HRT in perimenopause has been shown to provide greater symptom relief and support brain health in the long term.

Cautions

The risks of HRT will be unique to you as they vary based on your age, medical history and family's medical history, along with the type and duration of treatment. It is important to bear in mind that HRT is not usually effective at controlling heavy menstrual bleeding which can be a problem for some women and lead to other problems like iron deficiency from blood loss. It also does not act as a contraceptive. Yes, you can still conceive while you are ovulating in perimenopause.

With some forms of HRT, there is a slight increase in the risk of breast and ovarian cancer. This risk typically increases if taken for longer but falls after it is ceased. You should discuss this with your doctor, as your risk level is very individual, and there are strategies your doctor can employ to reduce risk. There are also some circumstances where increased breast cancer risk is not so much of a concern. For example women who have had a hysterectomy and use oestrogen only HRT, experience little to no increased risk of breast cancer. In addition, use of vaginal (topical) oestrogen has not been shown to increase breast cancer diagnosis.

On the flip side, there are also potential benefits of HRT that go beyond symptom relief. While I've absolutely seen a vast improvement in quality of life for many women, there are other potential upsides. For instance, HRT helps prevent osteoporosis which can have major health impacts in later life. In addition, combined or oestrogen-only HRT may be associated with a lower risk of colorectal cancer. As you can see, it is a balancing act that you should discuss with your doctor.

The pill

I often see women prescribed the pill during perimenopause to help regulate hormones and heavy and/or irregular periods. The pill is usually very effective at this, providing fast and effective relief from many hormonal symptoms. It's particularly useful if iron deficiency is a concern due to excess blood loss. The pill delivers a steady, level dose of hormones to suppress ovulation and regulate the cycle. There are some key things to be aware of. The pill usually contains higher doses of synthetic hormones such as ethinyl estradiol and progestins. (Some brands in Australia use body-identical oestrogen.) Side effects include irregular vaginal bleeding, nausea, sore or tender breasts, headache, bloating, changes to your skin and mood disturbances. Taking the pill leads to a very small increase in the risk of deep vein thrombosis (a blood clot), heart attack or stroke. It may also lead to a very small increase in the risk of breast cancer. The pill reduces the risk of endometrial and ovarian cancer. Importantly, the pill may mask the arrival of perimenopause and menopause but not delay it as it does not support hormonal balance, but rather overrides the natural progression.

There are other contraception options, or options to control heavy periods, such as intrauterine devices, but these are best discussed with your doctor.

What else is there?
So, what do you do if, for some reason, you can't take HRT? Whether it's due to other medical conditions, or you simply don't tolerate HRT, some women aren't able to add this to their treatment plan. Of course, your doctor will guide you here, but it's good to be aware of some other options at your disposal.

A good example is **fezolinetant**, which is a once-a-day, non-hormonal therapy for vasomotor symptoms (hot flushes and night sweats) associated with menopause. This drug works to block receptors in the brain that help regulate body temperature. In a study of women aged 40-65 years with moderate to severe hot flushes, fezolinetant reduced the frequency of symptoms over a 12-week period. Although HRT tends to be more effective when it comes to hormonal symptom relief, this is a good option where HRT is not on the table. It can't be used for all women and may or may not be effective for you in perimenopause, so you need to check with your doctor if it's safe and suitable for you.

Like all things health, whether or not HRT, the pill or other treatments are right for you will be determined by yourself and your doctor. There are many nuances.

What about GLP-1s?
I have no doubt you've heard about glucagon-like peptide-1 receptor agonists (GLP-1s) for weight loss. They are taking the world by storm, and the topic is a full book in itself.

As weight gain and changes to body fat distribution are a common theme in perimenopause, I commonly get asked about their efficacy in this phase of life. At the time of writing this book,

LIFESTYLE SHIFTS THAT MAKE A DIFFERENCE

specific research in perimenopausal women is still emerging, so I can't comment on the science. There is research to show that in post-menopausal women, the use of these agents together with HRT is more effective for weight loss and metabolic health than using a GLP-1 alone. Speak to your doctor if you want to learn more.

SUMMARY OF LIFESTYLE TOOLS AND TACTICS

SUMMARY OF TACTIC	HELPS WITH	RELEVANT TO MY GOALS Y/N
Self-care and mindfulness Add some meditation and mindfulness activities to your day to promote calmness and feeling grounded.	Mood changes, increased stress, sleep disturbances, hot flushes, night sweats, aches and pains.	
Establish a sleep routine Stick to a sleep schedule. Be aware of the impacts of food, drinks and exercise on sleep. Create a restful environment. Unplug before bed. Feast your eyes on morning sunlight for better sleep!	Sleep disturbances, low energy levels, brain fog.	
Regular exercise Include strength (resistance) training at least 2-3 times a week. Short bursts of cardio are ideal. Daily movement for the win. Balance it all out.	Muscle and bone health, heart health, low energy levels, sleep disturbances, mood, weight control, hormonal symptoms.	

LIFESTYLE SHIFTS THAT MAKE A DIFFERENCE

SUMMARY OF TACTIC	HELPS WITH	RELEVANT TO MY GOALS Y/N
Limit endocrine disruptors in the home Minimise cosmetics, skincare and household products that contain phthalates and parabens. Limit exposure to endocrine-disrupting chemicals.	Hormonal fluctuations.	
Medical treatments HRT, the pill and others	Speak to your doctor about your options.	

Leverage your lifestyle choices

Want the great news? These wonderful lifestyle tactics benefit your health beyond the realm of perimenopause. Remember, this is just a life phase. You will spend much of your life out of perimenopause and by improving your lifestyle, you are setting yourself up for longer-term better health and wellness. In the vein of knowledge equals power, I hope you leave this chapter feeling hopeful and motivated. Who would have thought that lovely acts such as feasting your eyes on morning light, spending time in nature, moving your body more, adding in calming breathing techniques and choosing more natural cosmetic products could play a role in managing perimenopause symptoms. And at the same time, you now have the lowdown on medical treatment options which you can discuss with your doctor, so they can help you develop a plan of action from that point of view. A healthy lifestyle includes having an established GP to help keep your health in check.

That closes off our section on lifestyle tactics for perimenopause. While these tactics are certainly not exhaustive, they are ones I have found to help improve symptoms with my clients. They are a good launching pad when you are making small changes to reap the benefits, and when getting on the road to feeling like you again.

Time to move on to the wild world of supplements.

Clinical case: Melanie's momentum

*All case studies are based on real client experiences. Names and personal details have been changed for privacy.

Like many new clients, Melanie came to see me to work out how to shed some extra kilos. Since her mid-30s, she had gained around 10 kg and felt like it just kept piling on. Now in her early-40s, she wondered if she just had to accept her new size and shape, or if there was something she could do about it. In our initial consultation, I discovered that Melanie was significantly under-fuelling. Her daily food and drink intake were nowhere near that required for a woman in her 40s, and it's likely her body was craving nutrients and energy to power her day. Her diet consisted mainly of white bread, rice, salad and a side of protein. Snacks were minimal, and she almost never felt hungry. To make matters worse, last year she had a terrible case of pneumonia and was in hospital for a few days. It's left her feeling low on energy ever since. After her hospital stay, her exercise regime fell apart and she cancelled her gym membership. If she was lucky, she now walked around 2,000 steps a day. She recently purchased a walking pad to place under her desk in an attempt to boost daily steps.

While Melanie was hoping for a tailored meal plan from our time together, my recommendations were loaded with lifestyle changes that could help her feel better and achieve weight-loss goals at the same time. We also discussed that weight alone is not the only determinant of health. We decided her SMART goals were not only to lose weight, but also to gain more energy and vitality, being the more important of the two goals.

What did I recommend?

- Aim for 10,000 steps a day. This is just a goal. The idea is to get Melanie to do more incidental movement throughout her day. Working up from 2,000 to 10,000 could take time, but chipping away at this daily helps work towards that goal.

- Consider buying a weighted vest to wear while walking.

- Slowly work towards 2 days a week at a new gym or return to her old one.

- Actively increase protein and fibre intake and include peri-beneficial foods in her diet.

- Speak to her doctor about repeating some blood tests to ensure low energy levels were not due to something else, and to get a pulse on her current health status.

Chapter 5
SMART SUPPLEMENT STRATEGIES

• • • • • • • • • • • • •

The calm of silence in the house makes Sophia smile. While Chris and Zoe are out, it's time for a cuppa, some TV and maybe even an at-home facial. But just before she boils the kettle, Sophia picks up her iPhone to quickly check for notifications to see if anyone liked her latest post. Just a few snaps of her delicious dinner last night, followed by a show in town.

No notifications. Just a moment then to scroll through the feed. *What's everyone else doing on this rainy Sunday afternoon? Oh look, there it is again.* Another young, thin influencer promoting creatine. She really should order some. According to *'Tips by Tiffany'*, it helps you gain muscle and lose belly fat. Sophia makes a mental note to use the TIFF10 code when she eventually places her order.

Next up, a woman gobbling down a stick of butter, and showing a day of eating in her world. *Carnivore diet*, she says, *it's all the rage*. Sophia wonders how they all seem to eat perfect food every day. They must be single. And childless. She scrolls on. A few happy snaps from her neighbour Amanda who is in Thailand for the week. Looks like bliss.

Ah, here we go. A woman who looks just like Sophia, probably around 40, holding a pink bottle of supplements. The headline reads 'banish perimenopause for good!' *This sounds promising.* These are the supplements Renee from the office mentioned. Apparently, they have helped so many women in her circle with hormonal issues. Renee said her mood swings and brain fog have virtually disappeared. Stuff it, Sophia thinks. ADD TO CART.

• • • • • • • • • • • • •

No doubt you are being inundated with reels, posts and stories about creatine, ashwagandha and magnesium for perimenopause. It's no surprise that Sophia is confused. Many of my clients feel the same way. So, where do supplements fit into this equation? How do they help with perimenopause, and do you need them? How do you choose the right ones and who can you ask for help? Strap yourself in. This section includes golden nuggets from my 20-plus years of experience in this industry. After reading it, I hope you never look at the label of a supplement or 'superfood' the same way ever again. And that's a good thing for your health – and your pocket.

In my clinic, I usually discover clients taking a range of supplements they have heard about, read about or been recommended in some way, shape or form. It's not uncommon for me to recommend they stop most of them. Now, don't get me wrong, I am a big advocate for supplements. But only if they have a specific need and are making a noticeable difference. Otherwise, you could find yourself on a weird concoction of supplements that interact badly with each other or your medications, and don't provide any real benefits.

3-step process to supplements

It can be hard to know what supplements you need, especially when you're being targeted with marketing and well-meaning acquaintances' recommendations. It probably goes without saying, speak to a health professional for specific advice on your unique circumstances. However, you can also use this simple 3-step process to analyse your supplement needs.

TIP

You may like to pause for a moment to take stock of what you are currently taking and see how they fit within this framework.

Step 1

KNOW YOUR BLOODWORK

In Chapter 2, we covered the importance of an annual blood test, and what tests to speak with your doctor about. The first port of call with supplementation is to rectify any issues found in your blood test results. For example, low iron may require supplementation. In this step, it's likely your doctor is also exploring the cause of such deficiencies. If not, you can always ask the question. Finding the root cause is essential. For example, iron deficiency may be due to heavy menstrual bleeding which can occur over long periods of time. Addressing this may negate the need for supplementation to a degree.

Step 2
ALLEVIATE SPECIFIC SYMPTOMS

Your bloodwork is now all considered. But you still have brain fog, trouble sleeping, night sweats and more. Here is where you can try specific, evidence-based supplements to see if they make a difference. I usually recommend trying one new remedy at a time, otherwise how do you know what has actually worked? Give a new supplement a try for 4-6 weeks, and if you do not feel a noticeable difference, go back to the drawing board.

Step 3
SUPPORT YOUR BODY IN THIS TRANSITION

Symptoms aside, there is a lot happening in your body at this time. Many of these changes cannot be seen or felt, but they are affecting your operating system. General supportive supplements may be helpful during perimenopause to help your body manage these changes, while also thinking about longer-term complications such as osteoporosis and heart disease.

> **BOTTOM LINE:** You don't always need supplements in perimenopause. But for some people, they can help support the body, overcome symptoms and prevent longer-term diseases.

Food or medicine, can you trust the claims?

In Australia, products sold as 'supplements' can either be classified as a food (e.g. bone broths, greens powders, manuka honey) or therapeutic goods, like multivitamins and herbal medicines to help treat or prevent symptoms or conditions. Why does this matter? The claims companies make about foods are typically much different to those of a therapeutic good. Foods generally have lower-level claims, such as a 'good source of calcium', whereas therapeutic goods can make higher-level claims such as 'assist in the prevention of osteoporosis'. While the nuance is often subtle, there is a reason why you should be aware of the difference.

It can also be confusing. For example, some foods are permitted to have specific nutrition, health or even higher-level claims, so always ask your health professional if unsure.

Therapeutic goods are held to higher standards and tend to have higher levels of active ingredients per dose. The thing is, there are fewer regulations for companies selling food. If I was launching a new superfood supplement, I would do all I could to avoid making it a therapeutic good. Then, I would use clever marketing to convince you to use my product for therapeutic needs, without stating it. Let's use an example to make this easier to spot. Keep in mind that this is general in nature to paint the picture in a very confusing market, so there are always grey areas.

Imagine I want to launch a herbal tea that has ingredients to help you sleep. As a food, I generally cannot state on the label that this tea is designed to help you sleep (a therapeutic claim). But, I can call the tea 'bedtime tea' and include images of a bed and some relaxing scenes on the label so that you associate this product with a sleep remedy. Truth be told, the amount of the herb you get from one cup of this tea is pretty unlikely to have a significant therapeutic effect. So, it is probably just a nice cuppa.

> **TIP**
>
> You can spot therapeutic goods pretty easily in Australia. Look for an AUSTL or AUSTR number on the label.

A word of caution

If you have any medical conditions or take other supplements or medications, be aware that some supplements won't mix well for you. Even certain foods and supplements don't agree with each other, and some perform better or produce fewer side effects (such as stomach upsets) when taken with food, or without. Although you may think supplements are always safe because you can buy them so easily, there are some cautions and warnings to be aware of, and not all are intended for long-term use. I have included safety tips in the section below for your reference, as well as some possible side effects. **These are general in nature and not exhaustive.** In any case, you should speak to your doctor before changing or commencing any new supplements to make sure they are suitable for you. And if you experience any suspected side effects, you should contact your doctor as soon as possible.

Common perimenopause supplements unpacked

In the next section, I have broken down some common perimenopause supplements under four headings: general supportive supplements, hormonal symptom support, energy support and stress, sleep and mood support. As science catches up, the majority of research in this space is in post-menopausal women. However, there is still relevance when relating to symptoms that are common in perimenopause, such as hot flushes. As the years go by, I have no doubt we will see more specific research into perimenopause.

While I have not dived into every ingredient that proposes to support this phase of life, I've chosen the ones I have seen most success with for my clients. If you are interested in other ingredients, I'd love to hear from you over on my social channels, so that I can share more with you in that forum.

General SUPPORTIVE SUPPLEMENTS

These are the supplements I've coined as the foundations of the house. Depending on your symptoms, perimenopause stage and other personal circumstances, each of these can play a different supportive role for many areas of your body and health.

Probiotics

HELPS WITH: Mood changes, hot flushes, night sweats, gut health, weight control, low energy levels, brain fog.

Changes to your gut health play a role in perimenopausal hormonal symptoms. In Chapter 3, you learnt all about nourishing your gut with specific foods. If you have trouble including enough fermented foods, prebiotics and probiotics in your diet, you can opt to have these in a supplement form. I must say, I do prefer a food-first approach to this, but it's not always possible to pack all the goodness in consistently. When it comes to probiotic supplements, there are specific types that may help more so with perimenopause symptoms. The key is to choose a product that contains the right strains of probiotics to optimise gut health, while helping with things like hot flushes, night sweats and mood swings. Not all probiotic strains are the same, and all have different effects on gut health and connected systems.

A group of probiotics known as lactic acid bacteria (LAB) has been shown to help alleviate hormone-related symptoms, such as low mood, hot flushes and night sweats. Although more research is needed in this space, including these in your regime could be supportive and help play a role in alleviating symptoms. LABs for these hormonal-related symptoms include *Lactobacillus rhamnosus*, *Lactobacillus acidophilus*, *Lactobacillus gasseri* and *Lactobacillus reuteri*.

The use of probiotic supplements may also help when it comes to weight control, much like the benefits when including probiotics in the diet. *Lactobacillus* and *Bifidobacterium* strains in particular show good results when it comes to weight reduction. When searching for a probiotic supplement, check the ingredient panel to be sure you're getting the right strains for perimenopause health.

> **TIP**
>
> You may find these LABs in probiotic supplements targeted towards women's health.

Possible side effects: Temporary gas or bloating, which usually subsides in a few weeks.

Safety tips: Not to be used if you have a condition that compromises your immune system, lymphoma, short bowel syndrome, severe pancreatitis or if you are taking corticosteroids as a long-term treatment.

Omega-3s

HELPS WITH: Heart health, brain fog, mood changes.

When it comes to supporting brain health and mood, as well as helping keep your cholesterol levels in check, omega-3s have an abundance of benefits. As you learnt, you can get these through foods, with the best options being fatty fish, like salmon and mackerel.

Let's recap the benefits of including omega-3s in your regime:

- May help increase levels of good cholesterol and reduce levels of triglycerides (a blood fat).
- Reduction in joint pain due to lowering inflammation in the body.
- Improvement of brain function and supporting a healthy mood.
- There is even a small study that showed omega-3s may help some women with night sweats.

Not all omega-3 supplements are created equal. When it comes to finding a good quality supplement, you should look for a product that:

- Contains both EPA and DHA, the types of omega-3 fats that have been shown to have specific health benefits.
- Contains a fish oil from a sustainable source and ideally with third-party certifications to attest to freshness, purity and the absence of any unwanted contaminants such as heavy metals or pesticides.

Fish oil supplements are a great option if you don't eat fish but are still open to consuming fish products. If you are considering plant-based omega-3 supplements, bear in mind that these are not as effective as animal-based ones (that contain EPA and DHA) and you may need to look at other tactics and/or supplements for added support. However, depending on your preferences, there are also algal oil forms of omega-3 supplements available. This oil is from marine algae, which can be rich in EPA and DHA, and boasts many of the same benefits as the fish versions of these ingredients. Ensure you choose a product that contains both EPA and DHA if you are going down the algal oil path.

Dose: The recommended daily omega-3 intake for healthy women is 1,100 mg. When it comes to supporting heart and cholesterol health, brain health and mood, doses can range from 1,000–4,000 mg per day. Take some time to check with your doctor, pharmacist or other health professional about what specific dose is best for you.

Possible side effects: Fishy or unpleasant taste, bad breath, headache and stomach upset.

Safety tips: Omega-3s can increase blood clotting time, so must be used under your doctor's supervision if you are taking blood-thinning medicines. Higher doses over extended periods of time may increase the risk of irregular heart rhythm (atrial fibrillation). Check with your doctor if you are concerned. If you have a fish or shellfish allergy, you must consult with your doctor. It is still unclear if fish oil supplements with omega-3 can cause reactions.

Collagen

HELPS WITH: Skin, bone and joint health.

Collagen, a naturally abundant protein in the body, provides structural support in connective tissue, muscle and skin. It accounts for around 30 percent of the whole-body protein content and plays an important role in skin elasticity, joint and bone health. The human body creates collagen naturally, and production declines with advancing age. Your body makes collagen from amino acids found in protein sources in your diet. In perimenopause, as oestrogen declines, this also contributes to a loss of collagen. So, what are the benefits of a collagen supplement in this life phase?

Skin health
Collagen has been shown to improve skin elasticity, which can help reduce fine lines and wrinkles.

Bone and joint health
We've covered how bone loss accelerates in perimenopause. Collagen can help increase bone mineral density, keeping bones healthy and strong. Research on athletes and people with osteoarthritis also suggests collagen may reduce joint pain.

Which source of collagen is best?
The main types of collagen found in supplements are derived from bovine species or marine life. There are some vegan products that contain the amino acids and nutrients the body needs to form collagen, but collagen itself is only found in animal sources.

When choosing a collagen, your best bet is to opt for a product that is labelled as hydrolysed collagen. This means the particles are smaller and easier for the body to absorb. Marine and bovine collagen have similar benefits, and some specific trademark collagens have researched benefits for skin, bone and other effects. Ask your health professional if you want to learn more. Vegan forms are not as well researched but do not seem to have the same benefits.

Dose: A dose range of 2.5 to 10 grams of collagen daily seems to be appropriate when it comes to some of the main benefits. You may like to choose a supplement that contains both collagen and vitamin C. Why? Vitamin C can help your body better absorb collagen supplements and enhance body collagen synthesis.

Possible side effects: Collagen supplements are well tolerated, but they may cause stomach upsets for some people.

Safety tips: Take care if you have allergies or sensitivities to certain sources (e.g. fish).

Magnesium

> **HELPS WITH:** Low energy levels, mood changes, sleep disturbances, hormonal symptoms.

Magnesium supports the body in a wide range of processes. It is an abundant mineral in the body, with various benefits for perimenopause. Magnesium plays a role in energy production, nerve and muscle health, mood balance, sleep quality, bone health, hormone balance, blood sugar control and blood pressure regulation. You can probably already see the connection to perimenopause symptoms that it may help manage. Many of the benefits of magnesium can be enjoyed through eating a range of whole foods such as wholegrain breads, green leafy vegetables, fruit (e.g. bananas, dried apricots), tofu, soy milk, yoghurt, avocado, legumes, nuts and seeds (e.g. pumpkin seeds, chia seeds). However, many people find magnesium supplements make a noticeable difference for specific symptoms, so you can trial it and see if it helps you.

Which type of magnesium is best?

Magnesium comes in a range of different forms. Limited research suggests that the different forms have different actions in the body. While more research on this is needed, there are some common examples to be aware of:

Sleep and relaxation

Magnesium glycinate, or magnesium bisglycinate, are highly absorbable forms of magnesium attached to a glycine molecule. Glycine has been shown to calm the brain, support better sleep and promote relaxation. As such, products with these forms of magnesium are promoted for their calming properties.

Brain health and focus

Magnesium L-threonate has been shown to help with memory and focus. It may even be promising when it comes to helping support a healthy mood. This form of magnesium crosses the blood-brain barrier, meaning it increases levels in the brain and neurons to exert its effect.

Period pain and PMS

A study showed that a 300 mg daily dose of magnesium helped relieve symptoms such as cramps, headache, back pain, irritability, and abdominal pain. For some women, menstrual pain can worsen in perimenopause, so this certainly holds some promise. Specifically, the **magnesium stearate** form was found to be most effective in this regard.

Dose: Women aged over 31 years should aim for 320 mg of magnesium per day. A tip is to check the amount of 'elemental magnesium' per dose, as sometimes the dose is expressed as the total chelated amount e.g. magnesium plus glycinate. You will also get some magnesium through food, so consider the 320 mg as an upper dose, if you like.

Possible side effects: Usually well tolerated but may cause stomach upsets for some people e.g. nausea, vomiting, diarrhoea. Go slow and gradually increase the dose to minimise this.

Safety tips: Should be used with caution in cases of kidney (renal) failure or diagnosed neuromuscular diseases.

Creatine

HELPS WITH: Muscle health and strength, brain fog, mood changes.

When it comes to sports supplements, creatine is up there with the most popular. And there's a good reason why. Creatine is an amino acid naturally produced by the body and stored in your muscles as an energy source for high-intensity explosive exercises. It is used as a supplement to boost muscle strength and athletic performance. During perimenopause and midlife, creatine supplements can help maintain muscle mass and strength. There is also research to show that creatine may help improve mood and cognitive function. When choosing a creatine supplement, look for one that contains 5 grams of creatine monohydrate per dose in a format that suits you best (e.g. powder, gummies, etc.). Choose brands with minimal additives where possible.

Possible side effects: You may hear that taking creatine can cause fluid retention or weight gain. Creatine can cause bloating and fluid retention for some people. It can sometimes cause temporary weight gain due to increased water retention. Keeping well hydrated while you are using creatine may help alleviate some of the side effects. If you cannot tolerate it, please speak with your doctor or pharmacist to see what's best for you.

Safety tips: Should be avoided if you have kidney disease.

Iodine

HELPS WITH: Breast pain, mood changes, weight control.

Iodine, an essential mineral, plays a role in various bodily functions, especially when it comes to thyroid health. Iodine has anti-oestrogenic effects, being helpful for perimenopause symptoms related to excess oestrogen, such as breast pain, and PMS-type mood changes. Iodine may also support metabolic health and weight control. This can be really helpful in some cases, but the dose needs to be carefully decided by your doctor, and specific directions and cautions apply, so please open the discussion at your next appointment if you'd like to learn more. Most of your iodine intake will come from your diet, through sources such as seafood (e.g. tuna, sardines), seaweed, dairy products, commercial bread, eggs and other foods with iodised salt.

Possible side effects: Stomach upset, headache, metallic taste in the mouth.

Safety tips: Just like all supplements, iodine is not suitable for all women and taking it without a thorough examination by your doctor could cause more harm than good. It can interact with other medicines or supplements.

A note on calcium and vitamin D

You already know all the bone-strengthening benefits of calcium and vitamin D in perimenopause from Chapter 3. While it's always best to get these through food or sunlight, there may be times when supplementation is best. Whether your doctor finds low levels in your bloodwork, you don't eat enough of these foods in your diet, or you have limited safe sun exposure, there may be a case for supplementation. This one is definitely for a discussion with your doctor to see what's right for you. You may be thinking, why don't I just take a supplement in case? Too much calcium or vitamin D may cause complications and unwanted symptoms.

If you do take a calcium or D supplement, choose one that contains vitamin D3 plus vitamin K2. Why? Once you reach menopause, your risk of heart disease increases. A buildup of calcium in the arteries may be a sign of possible blockages coming, and a higher risk of heart disease. That's why in menopause you should get your coronary artery calcium (CAC) test done, to know your level of risk, and take relevant actions. Here's where K2 comes in handy. It helps transport calcium to your bones, which need extra support to stay strong in this phase of life, while reducing the amount that ends up in your artery walls. And all the while, vitamin D increases calcium absorption. This is the ultimate trio!

Hormonal-symptom SUPPORT SUPPLEMENTS

While many perimenopause symptoms can be linked to hormone changes, there are some that can be particularly troublesome, such as hot sweats, mood changes and even midline weight gain. This set of supplements will play a role in supporting hormonal changes in midlife.

Your naturopath should be your best friend, especially in midlife, as there are many wonderful herbs that may make a difference when it comes to hormonal symptoms. Included in this section is a snapshot of some of the most common herbal remedies, but your best bet is to find a naturopath who can provide specific guidance. Err on the side of caution when looking to purchase a natural remedy for symptoms, as you will see below that research can be somewhat limited. But also remember each person has a different experience, so there may be merit in trialling some ingredients if you have not had much success with anything else.

Red clover (*Trifolium pratense* L.)

HELPS WITH: Hormonal symptoms such as hot flushes.

Red clover contains isoflavones, a type of phytoestrogen shown to bind to oestrogen receptors in the body, theoretically mimicking the effects of oestrogen. Studies show that it may be helpful in the short term for hot flushes during pre (or early) menopause for some people, but results are varied, and long-term effects have not been clearly demonstrated. The typical dose for hormonal symptoms is 40 to 80 mg per day of a product which is labelled to have standardised isoflavones.

Possible side effects: Red clover is usually well tolerated but may cause some vaginal spotting, skin irritation, nausea, headache and changes to the menstrual cycle (longer than usual periods).

Safety tips: As with phytoestrogens found in food, red clover should not be used in women with hormonal disorders, diagnosed hormone-sensitive conditions such as endometriosis, or in those with oestrogen-dependent breast cancer, or risks of this.

Vitex (Vitex agnus-castus)

HELPS WITH: Hormonal symptoms such as hot flushes, night sweats and mood changes.

Also known as chaste tree or chasteberry, this is a Mediterranean shrub used for the treatment of perimenopause-related symptoms. Limited research suggests that taking this herb may lead to moderate improvements in symptoms such as hot flushes, night sweats and maybe even mood. The dose is not so clear cut for this one, so it's best to speak to your naturopath, but it usually varies from 3.2–40.0 mg per day.

Possible side effects: Reported side effects include nausea, headache, stomach upset and rash.

Safety tips: It is thought that like red clover, vitex possesses some phytoestrogens, so again, caution is to be taken with hormonal disorders or in those with oestrogen-dependent breast cancer or risks of this. It is not to be used if you have any diagnosed hormone-sensitive conditions, such as endometriosis. Vitex can also interact with medicines such as the oral contraceptive pill, or other medicines. Check with your doctor before trying this one, especially if you are taking other medicines or have a mental health condition or Parkinson's disease.

Evening primrose oil

HELPS WITH: Hormonal symptoms such as night sweats.

Another common remedy is evening primrose oil. The oil is extracted from the seeds of the evening primrose (*Oenothera biennis*) plant. While the science is still emerging, and some older research showed mixed results, newer studies suggest evening primrose oil may help relieve the frequency and duration of night sweats. The dose in this case was 1,000 mg twice daily.

Possible side effects: Evening primrose oil is usually well tolerated, but some people may experience abdominal pain, nausea or diarrhoea.

Safety tips: Be cautious about using evening primrose oil if you have a diagnosed bleeding disorder, seizure disorder or mania.

Black cohosh (*Cimicifuga racemosa* or *Actaea racemosa*)

HELPS WITH: Hormonal symptoms such as hot flushes and mood changes as well as joint aches and pains.

Black cohosh has been found to alleviate hot flushes and joint aches and pains for some women. In addition, it has a calming effect on the nervous system, helping support mood changes. As there is only limited research in this space, some evidence is inconclusive as to whether or not black cohosh is an effective option for symptom relief. For this one, make sure you speak to a naturopath to determine if it is a good option, and to access a quality product at the right dose for you. Doses typically vary from 40 to 128 mg per day.

Possible side effects: Reported side effects include breast pain or tenderness, irregular menstrual cycles, nausea and stomach upsets.

Safety tips: Black cohosh has been reported to cause some serious cases of liver damage, but it is unclear how often this occurs. It may not be safe for women who have had hormone-sensitive conditions such as breast or uterine cancer. It should not be used by women who take the drug called tamoxifen.

Siberian rhubarb (Rheum rhaponticum)

HELPS WITH: Hormonal symptoms such as hot flushes.

Rheum rhaponticum is a species of Siberian rhubarb that is native to areas of Siberia and northern China. It has been specifically studied for its ability to relieve symptoms of menopause. Research shows that a specific extract called ERr 731™ can provide some symptom relief, especially when it comes to hot flushes, while taking 4 mg over a 4-week period.

Possible side effects: Common reported side effects include skin irritation, rash and stomach upsets, e.g. diarrhoea, nausea, cramps, abdominal pains and bloating. It is, however, generally well tolerated.

Safety tips: Long-term use appears to be safe. *Rhaponticum* may increase the risk of kidney stones.

Wild yam cream

HELPS WITH: See below.

I am including this one here by exception as it is not one that has clear evidence of benefits based on current scientific research. However, with the rise of social media trends, it is one that has gone off the charts based on some viral videos. While there may be ingredients in wild yam cream that theoretically act like oestrogen in the body, there is little science to suggest it works for symptom relief. This ingredient can also be found in a supplement form, which also lacks substantive evidence at this time. Interestingly, body-identical hormone replacement therapy can be derived from wild yams, but it is then converted in a laboratory to the end version of hormones.

Energy SUPPORT SUPPLEMENTS

We've covered all the many reasons why you may feel a bit low on energy. While diet and lifestyle are great ways to address this, you may still find yourself in need of an additional boost. If so, here are some products to consider.

Iron

HELPS WITH: Low energy levels, brain fog.

When it comes to energy levels, we've discussed the importance of keeping an eye on your iron intake. But in some cases, diet alone is not enough to get your iron levels where they need to be for optimal health. For this one, it's best to get a blood test before you start supplements, as taking iron when you don't need it can cause other complications. My top recommendation when it comes to iron supplements is to choose a product that contains *iron bisglycinate*, a very absorbable form that also tends to be gentler on the stomach. Your health professional can help you select the best dose.

Taking iron supplements with vitamin C tablets or orange juice can enhance absorption. However, it is best to separate the dose from certain foods, which can pair with the iron and reduce its absorption. Try to avoid the following foods and drinks for one hour before or two hours after taking iron supplements: dairy foods, eggs, spinach, tea, coffee or wholegrain breads. You should not take iron supplements and antacids or calcium supplements at the same time. Space doses one to two hours apart to get the full benefit from each.

Possible side effects: Gastrointestinal side effects are usually the most common concern with these supplements (e.g. constipation, stomach upsets). This can be minimised by taking iron supplements with meals. Start at a lower dose and gradually increase with alternate-day dosing, as the absorption can actually be higher when taken this way.

Safety tips: Liquid iron supplements may stain the teeth, so are best taken using a dropper that is directed to the back of the throat. If you have a blood disorder or take other medicines consult your doctor before starting iron supplements.

B vitamins

HELPS WITH: Low energy levels, brain fog.

Vegetables, fruits, whole grains, lean protein sources, dairy and fruit. What do these all have in common? They are all rich in B vitamins, and if you ask me, I'd rather pack more of this goodness into my day than add another supplement to the regime. However, sometimes you may be travelling, busier than usual or for some reason, feeling like you just aren't eating as much of these as you'd like. Or you may find out you have a deficiency via blood test results. If you follow a vegetarian or vegan diet, you will likely have to supplement with B12, as this is mainly found in animal foods. Some plant-based milks, cereals and meat substitutes can be fortified with B12. Another good source of plant-based B12 is nutritional yeast – this is a great way to add flavour to soups and casseroles, too.

If after considering all of that, you need to add a B supplement to your day, here's what you need to know. Bear in mind that research does not show that taking B supplements necessarily boosts energy for everyone who takes them. The greatest impact will usually be seen with a known deficiency. There are actually thirteen B-group vitamins in the body that all work together to support a variety of processes. Vitamins B1, B2, B3, B5, B6, B7, B9 and B12 are the specific types that help support and maintain energy levels and vitality. The way these vitamins support energy levels is varied, but on the whole, they help with energy production through assisting metabolic processes. You can buy what is called a B-complex vitamin supplement, which generally has these eight B vitamins in one tablet or capsule. The dose required can be specific to your needs, so best to speak to a doctor or pharmacist to be sure what you have selected is right for you.

Possible side effects: Taking more B vitamins than you need may lead to a variety of unwanted effects. For example, if you take too much B6, you may end up with excess levels in the blood, causing symptoms such as burning, tingling, itching and nerve damage. Other side effects may include bright yellow urine, stomach upset and headache.

Safety tips: Many products contain B vitamins which are listed with different names. Be careful not to double up. Just like with B6, there can be complications if you take too much of any one B vitamin. Alternate names to look for are:
- Thiamin (vitamin B1)
- Riboflavin (vitamin B2)
- Niacin (vitamin B3)
- Pantothenic acid (vitamin B5)
- Pyridoxine (vitamin B6)
- Biotin (vitamin B7)
- Folate (vitamin B9)
- Cobalamin (vitamin B12)

Stress, sleep and MOOD-SUPPORT SUPPLEMENTS

The intersection of perimenopause with other major life events, like changing family schedules, ageing parents and busy work lives, means women often feel a heavy burden. Managing stress, sleep and mood might need some extra attention in some cases, with specific supplements.

Ashwagandha (Withania somnifera)

HELPS WITH: Hormonal symptoms, stress and sleep disturbances.

An Ayurvedic herb, ashwagandha is a well-known remedy for stress and sleep. It belongs to a group of herbs known as adaptogens, meaning it helps the body better adapt to and resist physical and mental stress. A research study showed that this herb also helped some women with hormonal symptoms of perimenopause, such as hot flushes and urinary symptoms. Ashwagandha may even reduce perceived stress and anxiety and improve the quality and duration of sleep. The main way it is thought to work is by lowering levels of cortisol to help regulate the natural stress response. A common dose for anxiety and stress is 300 mg of ashwagandha root extract taken twice daily. In my clinic, women have found ashwagandha to be effective, but it may not be the ultimate solution for all cases.

Possible side effects: There have been some cases of liver damage (and liver failure), brain fog, worsened depression and altered behaviour when taking ashwagandha. This was usually seen at higher doses of around 900mg or above. Always seek advice from your health professional before trialling. Other reported side effects include drowsiness, stomach upsets, diarrhoea, and vomiting.

Safety tips: Best not used for extended periods of time. Ashwagandha appears to be most safe when taken in the short term (up to 3 months). If you have a diagnosed autoimmune disease (e.g. lupus), rheumatoid arthritis, type 1 diabetes or Hashimoto's thyroiditis, you are best to avoid ashwagandha.

St John's wort (*Hypericum perforatum*)

HELPS WITH: Mood changes, hot flushes.

St John's wort is a flowering plant of European origin that has been used to treat mild to moderate depression and low mood for many years. This plant contains many chemical compounds which are thought to increase the level of chemical messengers in the brain, such as serotonin. Various research papers suggest that its use for menopausal symptoms has merit when it comes to alleviating low mood, as well as reducing the frequency and severity of hot flushes. The dose of this one varies somewhat in the literature when it comes to menopause benefits, but in general, 900 mg per day (in divided doses) seems to be related to mood effects. Products will vary based on the specific active components they are standardised to contain, so it may be worth checking with your naturopath to be sure.

Possible side effects: Common side effects include stomach upset, diarrhoea, dizziness, dry mouth, fatigue, skin reactions after sun exposure, headache, insomnia, restlessness and sedation.

Safety tips: St John's wort can interact with many different medicines and other herbs or over-the-counter supplements. This can lead to negative consequences in some cases. It is also not suitable for use with specific diagnosed medical conditions such as bipolar disorder or schizophrenia. Always speak to your doctor before starting this herb. Long-term use and safety research is a bit limited so discuss this with your health professional.

Melatonin

HELPS WITH: Sleep disturbances.

Melatonin helps balance your normal sleep-wake cycle and resets your body clock to sleep and wake at the right times. You can boost your melatonin levels by spending daylight hours outdoors to expose yourself to natural sunlight, and by avoiding bright lights close to bedtime.

Before you go to bed, try drinking a cup of tart cherry juice which is rich in tryptophan and melatonin to help regulate sleep. Look for varieties with no added sugar. Or try a glass of cow's milk, or a handful of pistachios or cashews. You can also ask your pharmacist or doctor for melatonin tablets (which may be suitable for some people) to help you sleep better for longer.

Possible side effects: Melatonin tablets are generally well tolerated. May cause headaches, dizziness, nausea or daytime drowsiness for some women. If you feel drowsy, avoid driving, operating machinery or other such tasks.

Safety tips: Take caution when buying melatonin supplements. Some of these are homeopathic (highly diluted) or not well regulated, so you do not really know what you are getting inside the tablets, capsules, powders or gummies. Melatonin cannot be used with some diagnosed medical conditions and may interact with other medicines or supplements – always check before use.

SUMMARY OF COMMON SUPPLEMENTS

SUMMARY OF TACTIC	HELPS WITH	RELEVANT TO MY GOALS Y/N
General supportive supplements		
Probiotics	Mood changes, hot flushes, night sweats, gut health, weight control, low energy levels, brain fog.	
Omega-3	Heart health, brain fog, mood changes.	
Collagen	Skin, bone and joint health.	
Magnesium	Low energy levels, mood changes, sleep disturbances, hormonal symptoms.	
Creatine monohydrate	Muscle health and strength, brain fog, mood changes.	
Iodine	Breast pain, mood changes, weight control.	
Calcium, vitamin D and vitamin K	Bone health.	
Red clover, vitex, evening primrose oil, black cohosh, Siberian rhubarb	Hormone-related symptoms.	
Iron bisglycinate	Low energy levels, brain fog.	
B vitamins	Low energy levels, brain fog.	

SUMMARY OF TACTIC	HELPS WITH	RELEVANT TO MY GOALS Y/N
Ashwagandha	Hormonal symptoms, stress and sleep disturbances.	
St John's wort	Mood changes, hot flushes.	
Melatonin	Sleep disturbances.	

Time to reflect and move forward

I encourage you to take a moment here. We have covered a range of lifestyle and treatment options that can help you achieve your goals. You will not have to do every single one of these. Some will make sense for you as you work towards your SMART goals. Others will be good to know and be aware of but are not for adding in right now.

After reading Chapters 3, 4 and 5, you have a huge amount of new information that hopefully leaves you feeling empowered and in control when it comes to managing the symptoms of perimenopause. My hope is that you have filled your cup with evidence-based information that you can refer back to whenever you need. And when you hear an influencer, friend or colleague recommend a tactic they have used, you know you have your own tactics and soon-to-be Action Plan to guide you, while blocking out the background noise and confusion.

You are now ready to develop your Action Plan.

Clinical case: Olivia's overwhelm

*All case studies are based on real client experiences. Names and personal details have been changed for privacy.

Olivia was struggling with what she saw as a 'strange' group of symptoms impacting her quality of life. She shared with me the most troubling symptoms of aching joints, painful periods, intense bouts of anxiety, tingling hands and feet and midline weight gain. Olivia had been seeing a few practitioners to seek some relief, and felt things were not really getting any better. Upon review of her supplement regime, I discovered the following:

- She had 14 supplements in her plan. A mixture of ones to take daily, and a handful to use only as needed for specific symptom relief.

- Many of the supplements had duplicated ingredients.

- Olivia shared that she had new supplements added over time, and the list seemed to build up. Some of them, she just stored in her pantry as she wasn't even sure what they were for.

What did I recommend?

In this case, I reviewed all 14 supplements and pared them back to 5 key products that supported specific aspects of Olivia's health. Some of the ones we retained were un-opened, so had not yet been tried to see if they yielded symptom relief. I also ensured all formulations did not double up on ingredients, as I suspected the 4 products containing vitamin B6 could be contributing to the tingling in her hands and feet. We decided that Olivia would trial the new regimen for 4-6 weeks, along with nutrition and lifestyle tactics, to see how she felt, and what symptoms remained or dissipated.

Part III
FROM PLAN TO ACTION

I hope you are feeling ready to create your very own perimenopause Action Plan. You've done all the hard work at this stage, arming yourself with the knowledge about what's happening on the inside, then diving into nutrition, lifestyle and supplement solutions that will help you reach well-defined SMART goals.

The time has come to pair all your chosen tactics and propel you towards achieving healthy goals. And remember, this is a cyclical process. Go ahead and implement this Action Plan for 3-6 months. After you've given it a red-hot go, sit back and reflect, using the self-reflection tool provided.

Then come back, complete your self-assessment, and develop new goals. Then the process starts all over again. One thing's for certain. As you move towards the later stages of perimenopause, your symptoms will change. Some will go away, new ones will appear, and the cycle will continue. Your Action Plan process is always here to help you navigate new changes and guide you on science-based solutions to help you feel like you again.

PLAN
Self-assessment quiz
Set goals

PREPARE
Nail your nutrition
Level up your lifestyle
Demystify supplements

DO
Create an action plan
Reflect and repeat

Chapter 6
CREATE YOUR PERIMENOPAUSE ACTION PLAN

• • • • • • • • • • • • •

SOPHIA decides to go for a quick 15-minute jog. She's never been one for running, but it surprises her how much she enjoys slowly moving for 15 to 20 minutes around three times a week. It took a few weeks to find ways to move her body that she actually enjoys, and now it feels easy to keep up the routine. She giggles to herself as she hears the old 'A-Team' quote in her head *'I love it when a plan comes together'.* Gosh, Zoe would have no idea who The A-Team and Mr T are.

But seriously, she does love how this plan has all come together. She feels empowered with new knowledge about what her body is going through. And while she knows there are many tactics she can employ to feel better, she has a good grip on the nutrition, lifestyle and supplement tactics at her disposal, all of which are actually based on science!

A niggling voice in the back of Sophia's mind is wondering, *how will I keep all of this going, though?* It's so easy to fall off the bandwagon and settle back into old habits. Life throws curveballs, unexpected travel, illness and all sorts of things her way, but she really doesn't want to lose sight of why she started this journey. She wants to feel better and wave goodbye to these perimenopause symptoms that were getting more cumbersome over time. Surely there are some tips on sustaining her new lifestyle, because from what she's experienced thus far, the juice is worth the squeeze.

• • • • • • • • • • • • •

There's something about life that makes it hard to implement new things and actually stick to them. But rest assured, our friend Sophia is spot on when it comes to this side of it. There are ways to make it easier and more achievable in the long run. It's time to learn all about tips and techniques that help set you up for sustained success. Now there's no point sugarcoating it. In my clinic, this is by far the most challenging aspect when it comes to health. At this stage, my clients, and now you, have the foundational knowledge, and the tools and tactics they will implement to reach their goals. But what do you do when life throws you curveballs? We've all been there. That's when an Action Plan is non-negotiable in my book. On days when things don't go to plan, anchor yourself back to your Action Plan, and focus on what you can do to get back on track.

Health is a marathon, not a sprint

There is loads of science and research on why setting goals and creating a plan will improve your chances of success. But rather than deep dive into more science, I wanted to share a personal life experience that has taught me more about planning, goals, setbacks and more. And that's training for long-distance running. At the time of writing this book, I've completed one full marathon, and three half-marathon races. And while that makes me far from

CREATE YOUR PERIMENOPAUSE ACTION PLAN

a running expert, it does mean I've endured thousands of kilometres of training and all that comes with it. Without a plan, none of those races, and the ones to come, would ever be possible.

Here's what I've learnt, and why planning was absolutely critical at every stage of the journey:

- Big goals can seem unachievable at times. Like the hill ahead of you that has no visible peak, there are many opportunities to throw in the towel. The goal has to be something you genuinely want to achieve, otherwise there's little chance you'll keep going. And the goal needs to be tightly wrapped up into a plan so you can go back to the drawing board, reset and get back on track when you face setbacks.

- Setbacks are all part of the journey. All runners have had their fair share of injuries or soreness, wild weather conditions to contend with, or social functions that are right in the middle of a planned training session. I eventually accepted the notion that not everything will always go to plan. But I used my plan as a guide and made small adjustments to account for any unforeseen circumstances.

- Planning gave me a sense that I had more power over the future. By deciding in advance what I would do, when I would do it and how I would implement it, I had my own little mind map gently navigating me towards my end destination. It removed the worry, confusion and overwhelm that comes with committing to something like running 42.2 km in one go!

Planning is the secret sauce when it comes to achieving health goals. Just like training for a marathon, it helps set a path, lay the guardrails and create a framework that helps you implement the wonderful tools and tactics that will help you manage the symptoms of perimenopause.

Action Step
LET'S CREATE YOUR ACTION PLAN

It's time to connect all the dots and create your very own Action Plan. Using the template below (which is also available at my website), match your SMART goals with tactics across nutrition, lifestyle and supplements. Make any general notes about conversations you may like to have with your doctor in the space allocated.

Some tips when creating your plan:

- A good place to start is to refer back to the summary tables at the end of Chapters 3, 4 and 5. You hopefully completed these while the content from each chapter was fresh in your mind, and identified which tactics and tools best matched your goals.
- There is blank space for tactics in each area of nutrition and lifestyle and any supplements you may wish to try. There is no standard number of tactics you need in each area. It's unique to you.
- Remember, you don't need supplements, but there may be some you consider trialling based on your symptoms. Or some may be recommended by your health professional.
- I do recommend you include both nutrition and lifestyle tactics, as together these will support your body more holistically compared with just addressing nutrition or lifestyle alone.
- Be careful not to overcommit to too many new tactics, as this may cause overwhelm. Take a bite-sized approach and remember that you will come back to this step once you've spent 3-6 months adopting new practices.

- If you find it really easy to add your chosen tactics in, you can always come back at any time and add some more to your Action Plan. This is your journey, so you make the rules.

Perimenopause Action Plan

My SMART goal #1	
Nutrition tactics	
Lifestyle tactics	
Supplements	
Things to talk to my doctor about	

My SMART goal #2	
Nutrition tactics	
Lifestyle tactics	
Supplements	
Things to talk to my doctor about	

Be sure to head to http://www.thenutritionpharmacist.com/book-bonuses **to access your perimenopause Action Plan Template, self-assessment quiz, checklists, plus some additional bonuses that will support your journey further.**

Pillars for success

When working with women in my clinic, there are common themes when it comes to staying the course with your Action Plan. To help you succeed, I've compiled my top pillars for success and mindset cues that may support and guide you along the way.

Success pillar 1: Consistency is key

I can almost hear all my clients sigh as I say this annoying, but really important 'c word' – consistency. Now this has probably become my favourite word in the dictionary. When I think of consistency, it means staying the same at different times to the best of your ability and circumstances. This can help you form new habits and create behaviour change that leads to the actions you take every day. Being consistent most of the time is so much more important than perfection. Wow! So much to unpack right there!

Let's start with the end part. We're all human, so to expect perfection every single day as you show up and try to level up your health and wellness is unrealistic. Although it's great to set goals, and to plan your meals, exercise and wellness regime, you will have days where you cannot 100 percent stick to it. I have always travelled a lot for work, and some days I had no idea when my boss would stop for a meal, or what would be available for me. I always started those days with a realistic mindset and did what I could to control how my day panned out. I would pack nuts and seeds and healthy snacks. But sometimes I had to eat what I would have preferred not to and I had zero time to exercise. Did those days, or instances, which were less than 5 percent of my overall week, month or year, really have the potential to impact my health and wellness? No. I knew I consistently prioritised my health and wellness goals 95 percent of the time, and that's what matters most.

Success pillar 2: Your support crew

It always surprises me how many random strangers cheer you on in a marathon. People you've never met before do their utmost to get you across the finish line. While this is not to say random strangers will spur you on as you make changes to your lifestyle, having a support crew is a good place to start. You can share your plans and journey with trusted friends or family members and ask them to check in with you. You may like to choose an accountability buddy whom you can check in with every few weeks to update on your progress or status.

On your perimenopause journey, I cannot emphasise enough how important your health professional support crew will be. Your doctor, pharmacist, dietitian, nutritionist, naturopath, psychologist or other professionals will be guiding lights along the way. They can help bust myths, alter your plan based on your personal circumstances and offer you other treatment options only they can prescribe.

What does a naturopath do? Naturopaths take a holistic approach to health and wellness. They tend to focus on discovering the root cause of health problems versus simply curing any associated symptoms. They are experts in supplements, especially when it comes to herbal medicines which can be found in many over-the-counter products. A good tip is to make sure the naturopath you choose is registered with their appropriate association, such as the Naturopaths and Herbalists Association of Australia (NHAA).

Success pillar 3: Dealing with setbacks, overwhelm and failure

Over the years I have noticed that us women can be particularly hard on ourselves when it comes to health. Many of my clients have shared feelings of guilt, shame and disappointment when

CREATE YOUR PERIMENOPAUSE ACTION PLAN

they haven't followed my guidance or have been less consistent than they would have liked. Setbacks, less-than-perfect weeks, unexpected changes and the like will always be present in life. How can you reframe these moments as positive lessons rather than failures? Instead of dwelling on what didn't go to plan, forgive yourself and move forward. Focus back on your goals and why you want to achieve them. I've found that once you start to see how the changes make you feel, keeping to the plan becomes a lot easier. Lean on your support crew, share how you feel and try your best to regain some consistency.

> **If you are feeling really overwhelmed, have a low mood, or feel anxious or unsettled, don't hesitate to book in with your doctor or psychologist for more support.**

SELF-REFLECTION TOOL

After you've implemented new tactics, it can be refreshing to reflect on what has changed for you. Too often in life we jump from one thing to the next, and we don't take the time to reflect. It can be easy to focus on what didn't go well.

> *Have symptoms eased?*
> *Have new ones emerged?*
> *Have any of your tactics made such a difference that you can't imagine life without them?*
> *Have you started new supplements and decided they make no real difference?*

Using the self-reflection tool, take a moment to keep a record of it all. You can do this weekly, monthly or every few months, whatever works for you. After a few months, you may like to complete your self-assessment quiz again (see Chapter 2) and determine whether or not you need to adapt or create new SMART goals.

Be sure to head to http://www.thenutritionpharmacist.com/book-bonuses **to access the self-reflection tool, your Action Plan template, self-assessment quiz, symptoms checklist, SMART goal template, plus some additional bonuses that will support your journey further.**

Action Step
SELF-REFLECTION TOOL

What's worked well?

_____
_____
_____
_____

What has been a challenge for you?

_____
_____
_____
_____

How have you **felt** during times of setbacks or difficulties staying on course?

_____
_____
_____
_____
_____

Have your symptoms changed? (For better, worse or the same?)

_____

_____

_____

_____

Have any new symptoms appeared?

_____

_____

_____

_____

On a scale of 1-10 (1 being 'not very far at all' and 10 being 'I have reached my goal') how far have you come in achieving your SMART goals?

Goal 1 _____

Goal 2 _____

This tool is designed to help you also focus on the positives. You may have been too distracted or busy to notice that your mood changes have reduced or your energy levels have increased. If one or more of your symptoms has not changed at all, what other tactics can you add in to try to get further towards your goals?

Bringing it all together

We're almost at the end of our journey together. But your journey has only just begun. You now have a personalised perimenopause Action Plan to guide you using science-based solutions for your symptoms. Now it's time to get started, enjoying new and interesting meals, diving into lifestyle changes that will soothe your nervous system, and approaching your health providers with more confidence when it comes to asking for support on your perimenopause experience. I'm hopeful that you no longer feel overwhelmed with the multitude of information coming your way on new diets, supplements and fast fixes for health.

It's time to get started on your Action Plan.

Bonus Chapter
HOW TO BUILD A PERI-HEALTHY PLATE

Having all the know-how when it comes to nutrition and perimenopause is only half the equation. It's all well and good to know you need to eat more omega-3s, up your protein, boost your fibre and add in hormonal-balancing foods, but how do you actually build main meals and snacks that tick all the boxes? Many of my clients are keen on me creating a meal plan for them. While I am happy to provide a few sample days for structural guidance, I'm not a huge fan of prescribing detailed meal plans. Here's why.

While meal plans are handy, and they technically allow for no (or little) margin for error, I've found they are not overly helpful in the long run. After a while, I can guarantee you will find a meal plan restrictive, and you will likely need to have a nutritionist consultation every month for the rest of your life so it can be mapped out for you. This is not realistic, nor budget friendly. What is helpful are the tips and tactics you need to master to make changes to your dietary patterns in the long term. So, rather than focus on a master meal plan with you, I'd rather guide you on how to build a peri-healthy plate so you can use this in any situation. Think of your nutrition tactics as the kickstart for your engine. You will need to continue to add fuel and run the engine every day by building healthy plates consistently to achieve results.

How to build a
PERI-HEALTHY MEAL

Step 1: Choose ingredients

Smart carb grain source: Oats, soy-linseed bread, brown basmati rice, pulse pasta or soba noodles (tip: bulk out with veggie zoodles made from zucchini or carrot or cauliflower/broccoli 'rice').

Low GI fruits and veggies: Sweet potato, capsicum, broccoli, asparagus, mushrooms, zucchini, spinach, cauliflower, green beans, lettuce, cucumbers, celery, tomatoes, onion, eggplant, cabbage, apples, oranges, grapes, apricots, plums, kiwis, peaches, pears, nectarines.

Protein: Palmful size of cooked chicken, lean meat, fish (omega-3 rich varieties) or vegetarian/vegan options (tofu, tempeh, egg, legumes). Yoghurt, cottage cheese, ricotta. Aim for at least 20–30 grams of protein with each main meal.

> **TIP**
>
> Choose 200 grams of soy-based protein sources (e.g. tofu or tempeh) if phytoestrogens are recommended for you.

Step 2: Toppers, seasonings, must-haves to help alleviate midlife symptoms

Hot flushes: Add ground flaxseeds, sesame seeds or sunflower seeds, top with almonds or pistachios for extra crunch.

Low on energy or brain fog: Add whole grains and lots of fruit and veggies. Add extra virgin olive oil as a dressing and/or to cook with.

Aches and pains: Add ginger, turmeric or cayenne pepper to soups and sauces. Top yoghurt with blackberries or blueberries.

Moody: Add omega-3 oily fish, top with walnuts, flaxseeds, chia seeds, hemp seeds.

Gut-healthy essentials: Add sauerkraut, kimchi, pickles, miso, yoghurt and kefir (great for dressings).

Peri-healthy
BREAKFAST RECIPES

BREAKFAST EGG WRAPS

SERVES 1
PREPARATION 5 minutes
COOKING 5 minutes

2 × eggs
1 × low-GI wrap, preferably wholemeal
50 g cup cottage cheese (regular fat)
½ medium tomato sliced
Handful of spinach leaves
¼ avocado sliced
½ tsp extra virgin olive oil
1 tsp sriracha and kimchi (optional)

1. Beat eggs in a bowl, and season with salt and pepper to taste.
2. Wash and dry all your veggies, then prepare as required.
3. Heat oil in saucepan and cook eggs to your liking.
4. Get your wrap and place the eggs, tomato, greens, avocado, sriracha and kimchi on it, then wrap it all up your way.

Nutritional composition

	Per Serve
Energy	1849 kJ (442 cal)
Protein	27.9 g
Total Fat	20.3 g
Saturated Fat	5.75 g
Total Carbohydrates	31.7 g
Sugar	3.1 g
Dietary Fibre	8.9 g
Sodium	580 mg

APPLE AND BLUEBERRY PIE OVERNIGHT OATS

SERVES 2
PREPARATION 5-10 minutes

1 medium apple (any variety) peeled and grated
½ cup dry rolled oats
2 tsp chia seeds
1 tsp ground cinnamon
Pinch of salt
1 cup natural Greek yoghurt (approx. 240 grams)
1½ cups soy milk (can substitute for your choice of milk – choose an unsweetened variety of plant milk)
½ serve vanilla protein powder
¾ cup blueberries (wash and gently pat dry) plus extra for topping
Crushed pistachios as a topping

1. Combine well.
2. Place in an airtight jar or glass container.
3. Refrigerate for a few hours or overnight.

Double or triple the recipe and *batch this one!*

Additions

Top with fresh grated apple, blueberries and crushed pistachios for extra sweetness and crunch.

	Per Serve
Energy	1881 kJ (450 cal)
Protein	22.8 g
Total Fat	19.7 g
Saturated Fat	9.06 g
Total Carbohydrates	40.8 g
Sugar	24.5 g
Dietary Fibre	9.17 g
Sodium	264 mg

Peri-healthy LUNCH RECIPES

EASY NOURISH BOWL

SERVES 1
PREPARATION 5–10 minutes

½ cup cauliflower rice (heated) mixed with
    ¼ cup cooked brown basmati rice
Protein options: 1 × 95-gram can of tuna
    (BPA free) in olive oil, drained well or
    80 grams of cooked and shredded chicken (skin off)
1 cup spinach leaves
1 small can of beans (BPA free): 125 grams of
    edamame beans or 4 bean mix (drained well and rinsed)
½ tbsp extra virgin olive oil
2 tsp grated Parmesan cheese
Sprinkle of crushed walnuts to serve

1. Wash and dry all your veggies, then prepare as required.
2. Simply mix and serve!
3. Top with crushed walnuts.

Nutritional composition

TUNA	Per Serve
Energy	2233 kJ (534 cal)
Protein	34.0 g
Total Fat	25.2 g
Saturated Fat	5.10 g
Total Carbohydrates	38.60 g
Sugar	3.95 g
Dietary Fibre	11.4 g
Sodium	464 mg

CHICKEN	Per Serve
Energy	2080 kJ (497 cal)
Protein	38.3 g
Total Fat	19.1 g
Saturated Fat	4.40 g
Total Carbohydrates	37.9 g
Sugar	3.25 g
Dietary Fibre	11.4 g
Sodium	217 mg

PITA CHIPS AND CHICKPEA SALAD

SERVES 2
PREPARATION 10-15 minutes
COOKING 5 minutes

SALAD

1 x tin of canned chickpeas (BPA free), drained and rinsed well (approx. 400-gram can)
2 boiled eggs, chopped into small pieces
¼ red onion
2 Lebanese cucumbers diced
8 cherry tomatoes, diced
2 tsp extra virgin olive oil
Salt and pepper to taste

PITA CHIPS

1 medium wholemeal pita
Extra virgin olive oil spray (small amount)
Tip – choose a spray that does not contain any propellants like butane or propane.
1 tsp unhulled sesame seeds
150 grams cottage cheese (regular fat) to serve

1. Wash, dry and prepare veggies. Heat oven to 180°C.
2. Mix all salad ingredients together in a bowl.
3. Spray the pita bread with oil, sprinkle with sesame seeds, and bake in the oven for 5 minutes or until crisp. Break up as chips and serve.
4. Serve with a side of cottage cheese.

Nutritional composition

	Per Serve
Energy	2471 kJ (591 cal)
Protein	37.1 g
Total Fat	18.9 g
Saturated Fat	5.20 g
Total Carbohydrates	55.9 g
Sugar	10.9 g
Dietary Fibre	16.3 g
Sodium	1170 mg

Peri-healthy DINNER RECIPES

ZESTY PROTEIN PASTA BOWL

SERVES 2
PREPARATION 10-15 minutes
COOKING 15 minutes

80 grams dry protein pasta – spaghetti style works best
100 grams raw chicken breast, or 150 grams grated tofu
Tip: If using tofu, pat dry and press under a heavy object for a few hours prior to grating for a better texture and easier grating.
2 cloves garlic, crushed
2 zucchini spiralised
2 cups spinach leaves
100 grams crumbled feta
Juice of half a lemon
1 tsp extra virgin olive oil plus 1 tbsp for dressing
Salt and pepper to taste
2 tsp hemp seeds.

1. Cook pasta according to packet instructions.
2. While pasta is cooking, heat olive oil and cook tofu or chicken with garlic until cooked to your liking.
3. Wash and dry all your veggies, then spiralise zucchini and blanch (you can do this for the last minute of pasta cooking time, in the same pan).
4. Drain pasta and zucchini and mix through crumbled feta and cooked tofu or chicken.
5. Mix through lemon juice, spinach leaves and extra virgin olive oil.
6. Add salt and pepper to taste.
7. Top with hemp seeds.

Nutritional composition

CHICKEN	Per Serve
Energy	1948 kJ (466 cal)
Protein	34.2 g
Total Fat	24.3 g
Saturated Fat	9.88 g
Total Carbohydrates	24.1 g
Sugar	4.86 g
Dietary Fibre	7.5 g
Sodium	140 mg

TOFU	Per Serve
Energy	2190 kJ (523 cal)
Protein	32.11 g
Total Fat	31.3 g
Saturated Fat	10.7 g
Total Carbohydrates	24.1 g
Sugar	4.86 g
Dietary Fibre	10.1 g
Sodium	149 mg

SALMON AND EDAMAME NOODLES

SERVES 1
PREPARATION 5-10 minutes
COOKING 15-20 minutes

100 grams raw salmon (skin off)
2 tsp extra virgin olive oil
1 cup broccoli florets, chopped into small pieces
1 carrot, chopped into small pieces
¼ onion diced
2 cloves garlic, crushed
50 grams cooked soba noodles
1 tbsp reduced-salt soy sauce
1 tsp turmeric powder
1 tbsp sriracha
1 tsp unhulled sesame seeds

1. Heat the oven to 180°C.
2. Use 1 teaspoon of oil to coat salmon, season with salt and pepper, then bake in the oven at 180°C for 15 mins or until it's cooked to your liking.
3. Meanwhile, use the other teaspoon of olive oil to sauté onion and garlic, then add in other veggies and cook until soft. Add in sauces and turmeric and mix well. Add a little water to help steam and accelerate the cooking process.

4. Cook noodles according to pack instructions, drain, then add to the pan with the veggies and mix through.
5. Top with salmon and sesame seeds and serve.

Nutritional composition

	Per Serve
Energy	1928 kJ (461 cal)
Protein	25.4 g
Total Fat	24.9 g
Saturated Fat	4.69 g
Total Carbohydrates	29.2 g
Sugar	13.9 g
Dietary Fibre	8.9 g
Sodium	885 mg

Peri-healthy SNACK GUIDE

Step 1: Choose colours
Make your snacks as colourful as possible.

More colours equals more antioxidants and plant ingredients to fuel and protect your body.

Step 2: Choose protein
Healthy protein options: 100 grams of natural unsweetened yoghurt (high-protein varieties are even better), 1-2 teaspoons of nut butters, eggs, cottage cheese, hummus, protein powders.

Step 3: Choose toppings
Whole grains and/or healthy fats will help keep you satisfied and nourish your body. Use small portions of wholegrain muesli, chia seeds, or a sprinkle of nuts as toppers.

Peri-booster options

Phytoestrogen boosters: Ground flaxseeds, sunflower seeds, almonds, pistachios, pomegranates.

Calcium boosters: Dairy or calcium-fortified soy milk or soy yoghurt, cottage cheese, almonds, Brazil nuts.

Gut boosters: Remember that yoghurt and kefir are extra powerful for gut health – check for added probiotics on the label. Green bananas for resistant starch. Fermented foods like sauerkraut, kimchi and pickles.

Here are some examples to get you started

- Slice 1 medium green banana and serve with 1 teaspoon of almond butter spread evenly over each slice.

- 100 grams of Greek yoghurt, mix in ¼-½ scoop of vanilla or chocolate protein powder, add some crushed pistachios, plus a handful of berries.

- 2 wholegrain crackers topped with hummus, sliced tomato and some sunflower seeds.

- Mixed berries with yoghurt, topped with crushed almonds and Brazil nuts.

- 2 soy-linseed crackers with cottage cheese, and sliced tomato or cucumber. Add some sauerkraut to top.

- Yoghurt bark – mix 100 grams of yoghurt with a sprinkle of berries, pumpkin seeds, hemp seeds and a dash of honey. Freeze for 60 minutes (or overnight), break into pieces and keep stored in the freezer.

Hot flushes

In Traditional Chinese Medicine, foods are categorised as having cooling or warming properties. Although more research is needed, ancient remedies and modern research papers have explored this concept. When hot flushes strike, a relief strategy could be to eat or drink some cooling foods to help relieve that feeling of overheating and sweating that comes on oh-so-fast.

Cooling foods: Cucumber, radish, cabbage, bok choy, cauliflower, carrots, watermelon, pears and apples.

HOT FLUSH BUSTING SMOOTHIE

Blitz together (serves 1)
1 cup watermelon (frozen)
½ cup cucumber sliced
½ medium apple (peeled)
½ lime, juiced
¾ cup water
Handful of ice (optional)

Bonus tip: How do I stop the after-dinner cravings?

If you find yourself craving sweetness after dinner, my number one piece of advice is to ask yourself if you ate enough during the day. Firstly, it's OK to have something sweet after dinner if you feel like it. Why not opt for a healthier option that provides nutrients and sweetness at the same time?

Try pairing a few squares of chocolate with a palmful of nuts and berries as a nutritious and tasty sweet treat. To further address the root cause of this question, I'd like you to reflect on what you ate during the day.

Did you have a nourishing breakfast, with some added protein and fibre to help keep you fuller for longer?

Did you eat a nutritious and satisfying lunch and dinner, with some well-balanced treats and snacks in between?

Did you hydrate well throughout the day?

The most common reason you feel hungry or unsatisfied after dinner is that you probably didn't fuel your body adequately that day. Under-consuming food is really common in women, especially those who were raised in the 'low-fat era' (think the late 1990s). This has flowed through into adulthood in some cases. The first step to crushing the late-night cravings is to get your nutrition foundations nailed and ensure you are giving your body the energy and nutrients it needs to perform at its best and feel satisfied as the day comes to a close.

RECIPE NOTES

Please note that the recipes are written using Australian standard weights and measures. Use cups and measuring spoons for dry and solid ingredients and jugs for measuring any liquids. Tablespoon measures: I have used 20 mL (4 teaspoons) tablespoon measures. If you're using 15 mL (3 teaspoons) tablespoons, add an extra teaspoon of the ingredient for each tablespoon specified.

Nutrition information *is approximate and based on current Australian nutrition composition databases using common brands where required.*

Gas				
Celsius (electric)	Celsius (fan-forced)	Fahrenheit	Gas	Heat
180°	160°	350°	4	moderate

BEYOND THIS BOOK

• • • • • • • • • • • • •

Four weeks of annual leave incoming. Sophia smiles as she puts her out-of-office reply on. *Cook Islands, here we come!*

After what has been a hectic year, Chris surprised her and Zoe with a two-week holiday of island hopping, and she couldn't be more excited. Six months ago, this would have caused so much anxiety. Worrying about what bathers might still fit, how she'll handle her mood swings in small hotel rooms with no place to decompress, what to choose at the breakfast buffet. But after working through her Action Plan, implementing bite-sized changes, uplifting her lifestyle and adding in a few targeted supplements, things are feeling better.

As for the mass confusion and overwhelm, while she'd be lying to say it has disappeared altogether, it has definitely reduced. Sophia is so much more picky with who she chooses to follow on Instagram, and uses it more for staying connected with friends and family, and choosing the next trending fashion item. Her algorithm has almost stopped sending her magic supplements that will cure every perimenopause symptom that exists, thank goodness for that! But, she still hears her friends chat about it and some of the 'noise' remains in the background. She feels good that she has a reference guide to go back to, and science-based tactics and tools that have had a positive impact on her health.

By far her biggest mindset shift has been around doing things that are good for her body and health in the long run. No more fad diets, quick fixes or miracle cures. It's all about building healthy habits, adapting as her symptoms change and focusing on how she can live a healthier, happier life.

• • • • • • • • • • • •

Sophia has been on this ride with you, from front to back cover. Have you seen glimpses of yourself in Sophia? Could you relate? I certainly can, as just like you, I'm in the midst of my perimenopause journey. She has been my anchor while creating this book. After speaking with many women, helping many clients and hearing many stories, I have spent the last two years getting deeply inside Sophia's head as I have written this book. It is my genuine hope that I have tackled some of your burning questions, cleared confusion and given you a clear path forward.

Perimenopause comes with lots of change. Coupled with information overload, often inconsistent health advice and more solutions than you can possibly try, it can be a testing time. But in a way, we should be grateful for this. Five or ten years ago, very few people were openly talking about perimenopause and menopause. The other day, one of my friends referred to us as 'the lucky generation' as she'd silently suffered through this phase, which impacted her personal and professional life immensely. It's no doubt the additional exposure has led to more focus in all areas, such as emerging research, education for health professionals and support options for women as you experience these changes. However, this has caused a state of information overwhelm. Every day, women tell me they have no idea what to do to feel better, where to turn to or who to trust. New remedies, programs, books, podcasts and blogs appear every week, it seems. I wrote this book to help cut through the noise and make your life easier. To ensure science-based recommendations are coming your way if you so desire. You can see all the references for further reading at the back. Think of this book as a reference manual you can come back to and read cover to cover. The power is now in your hands. You can create an Action Plan to meet your specific goals. And you also have thought-starters when it comes to speaking with your doctor. This is a key part of the journey.

If I can leave you with one piece of advice, it is to choose your sources of information wisely. Reach out to qualified health professionals, particularly ones who have completed additional training in perimenopause, menopause or women's health. Take care with following general advice that comes from unqualified people.

Reaching menopause

I've deliberately kept the content in this book to the perimenopause phase. But it's not lost on me that almost a third of a woman's life can be in the post-menopause phase, remembering that menopause is just a point in time when your periods have stopped for twelve months in a row. Some of the recommendations will remain similar, but there are definitely nuances when it comes to post-menopause, so once you get there, please seek advice on that phase from a validated source. Rest assured, whatever stage you are at, there are millions of women feeling the same. If we help each other, no one should ever feel alone on this journey. For now, that's where I'll leave you. I'm confident you have smart tools in your toolbox and a structured way to bring it all together among everyday life. Thank you to all my clients, followers and to you, my readers. You inspire me every day and nothing beats the stories and feedback on how your lives have changed for the good. I invite you to follow along at my social media channels and sign up to my newsletter via my website.

I want to finish with a client testimonial that warms my heart every time I read it.

> "After having seen a few other nutritionists around Melbourne over the years, I've found Sarah to be the best. She has that unique combination of expertise (and lots of it), enthusiasm, and a warm personality that makes her a pleasure to work with. After making some tweaks to my existing diet, and adding some supplements, my issues reduced significantly, and my GP and I were really pleased with the results. I highly recommend Sarah, and I look forward to working with her again."

Yours in peri-health
Sarah xx

ACKNOWLEDGMENTS AND GRATITUDE

Putting pen to paper to write this book has been harder than I ever imagined. It has taken a village to get me here, and none of this would have been possible without some incredible family, friends and mentors.

I start by thanking my amazing husband, Kieren. From listening to my ideas and dilemmas, to propping me up when the process became a bit overwhelming and everything in between. Most of all, for always believing in me more than I believe in myself.

To my mum, Anna, who is my number one supporter as well as my very best friend. In the early stages, you told me just to 'go for it' and that spurred me to actually get words on a page and push through as we cared for our beautiful dog Hugo while going through his cancer treatment. I am eternally thankful.

To my gorgeous furry children. Hugo, who has crossed over the rainbow bridge, I'll forever miss you. Your pawprint is eternally imprinted on my heart, and I'll never forget starting this book to help anxiously pass the time while we awaited your return home after many rounds of radiation. Charlie, who is my little shadow, buddy and avid listener as I proofed some chapters out loud for a while there. Winnie for being the best relaxation aid a girl could wish for. And Shilo, mum's best friend. Thanks to my brother, Dean, for being the best uncle dogsitter there is.

To Simone, the best neighbour I'll ever have, and a driving force for this book's topic, theme and focus. Thanks for the chats, the guidance and the never-ending support. It means a lot.

To Gabs, Soumya and Kate for being my superstar reviewers, keeping me in check and helping ease my desire to share absolutely perfect information with my readers. And to all my mentors, colleagues, peers and friends who were so happy to help out, no questions asked.

To Natasha Gilmour, who saw my vision even more clearly than I did from the moment we first met. For helping me bring this book to life, but most of all, for being one of the kindest, caring humans I have ever come across.

To Kelly Irving and the Expert Author community, and Kerryn Harvey, my accountability buddy in this group. Without these wonderful people, I'm certain this book would not be with you today.

And finally, to my incredible clients. Helping you is my privilege. Thank you for choosing and trusting me.

REFERENCES

Introduction
https://www.balance-health.com.au/post/7-million-women-in-australia-are-in-peri-menopause-or-menopause

Michalski, C. A., Diemert, L. M., Helliwell, J.F., Goel, V., Rosella, L.C. Relationship between sense of community belonging and self-rated health across life stages. SSM Population Health. 12, 12, 2020. https://doi.org/10.1016/j.ssmph.2020.100676

Chapter 1
Becker, S., Manson, J. Menopause, the gut microbiome, and weight gain: correlation or causation? Menopause 28, 327–331 (2020). https://journals.lww.com/menopausejournal/abstract/2021/03000/menopause,_the_gut_microbiome,_and_weight_gain_.14.aspx

Better Health Channel. Menopause and weight. *Better Health Channel* (n.d.). https://www.betterhealth.vic.gov.au/health/conditionsandtreatments/menopause-and-weight-gain

Better Health Channel. Premature and early menopause. *Better Health Channel* (n.d.). https://www.betterhealth.vic.gov.au/health/conditionsandtreatments/premature-and-early-menopause

Cleveland Clinic. Night sweats. *Cleveland Clinic* (2022, June). https://my.clevelandclinic.org/health/symptoms/16562-night-sweats

Cleveland Clinic. Perimenopause. *Cleveland Clinic* (2024, August). https://my.clevelandclinic.org/health/diseases/21608-perimenopause

Denniss, E., Lindberg, R., Marchese, L. E., McNaughton, S. A. #Fail: the quality and accuracy of nutrition-related information by influential Australian Instagram accounts. International Journal of Behavioral Nutrition and Physical Activity 21, 16 (2024). https://ijbnpa.biomedcentral.com/articles/10.1186/s12966-024-01565-y

Eaton, S., Sethi, J. Immunometabolic links between estrogen, adipose tissue and female reproductive metabolism. *Biology* **8**, 8 (2019). https://doi.org/10.3390/biology8010008

December Endocrine Society. Plastics, EDCs & health: Authoritative guide. Endocrine Society (2020, December). https://www.endocrine.org/topics/edc/plastics-edcs-and-health#1

Endocrine Society. *Menopause*. Endocrine Society (2022, January). https://www.endocrine.org/patient-engagement/endocrine-library/menopause

Endocrine Society. *Reproductive hormones*. Endocrine Society (2022, January). https://www.endocrine.org/patient-engagement/endocrine-library/hormones-and-endocrine-function/reproductive-hormones

Grant, L. K., Coborn, J. E., Cohn, A., Abramson, M., Elguenaoui, E., Russell, J. A., Wiley, A., Nathan, M. D., Scheer, F. A. J. L., Klerman, E. B., Kaiser, U. B., Rahman, S. A., Joffe, H. Effect of experimentally induced sleep fragmentation and hypoestrogenism on fasting nutrient utilization in premenopausal women. *Journal of the Endocrine Society* **5** (Suppl 1), A774 (2021). https://doi.org/10.1210/jendso/bvab048.1575

Harper, J. C., Phillips, S., Biswakarma, R., Yasmin, E., Saridogan, E., Radhakrishnan, S. C., Davies, M., Talaulikar, V. An online survey of perimenopausal women to determine their attitudes and knowledge of the menopause. *Women's Health (Lond. Engl.)* **18** (2022). https://doi.org/10.1177/17455057221106890

Herrera, A., Nielsen, S., Mather, M. Stress-induced increases in progesterone and cortisol in naturally cycling women. *Neurobiology of Stress* **3**, 96–104 (2016). https://doi.org/10.1016/j.ynstr.2016.02.006

Jean Hailes for Women's Health. *What is perimenopause*. Jean Hailes (2025, April). https://www.jeanhailes.org.au/resources/perimenopause-fact-sheet#:~:text=About%2020%25%20have%20no%20symptoms,e.g.%20sore%20breasts%20and%20migraines

Karasek, M. Melatonin, human aging, and age-related diseases. *Experimental Gerontology* **39**, 1723–1729 (2004). https://doi.org/10.1016/j.exger.2004.04.012

Kim, D. R., Joffe, H. Use of antidepressants during perimenopause. *Women's Health* **2**, 627–637 (2006). https://doi.org/10.2217/17455057.2.4.6

Lo, J. C., Burnett-Bowie, S. A., Finkelstein, J. S. Bone and the perimenopause. *Obstetrics and Gynecology Clinics of North America* **38**, 503–517 (2011). https://doi.org/10.1016/j.ogc.2011.07.001

Magraith, K., Stuckey, B., Baber, R. Perimenopausal hormone therapy – Assessment and prescribing. *Medicine Today* **23**, 61–66 (2022). https://medicinetoday.com.au/mt/2022/august/regular-series/perimenopausal-hormone-therapy-%E2%80%93-assessment-and-prescribing

REFERENCES

Mayo Clinic. *Premature ovarian insufficiency*. Mayo Clinic (2023, October). https://www.mayoclinic.org/diseases-conditions/premature-ovarian-failure/symptoms-causes/syc-20354683

Mayo Clinic. *The reality of menopause weight gain*. Mayo Clinic (2023, July). https://www.mayoclinic.org/healthy-lifestyle/womens-health/in-depth/menopause-weight-gain/art-20046058

McCarthy, M., Raval, A. P. The peri-menopause in a woman's life: A systemic inflammatory phase that enables later neurodegenerative disease. *Journal of Neuroinflammation* **17**, 317 (2020). https://jneuroinflammation.biomedcentral.com/articles/10.1186/s12974-020-01998-9

Mumusoglu, S., Yildiz, B. Metabolic syndrome during menopause. *Current Vascular Pharmacology* **17**, 595–603 (2019). https://doi.org/10.3390/metabo12100954

Ryczkowska, K., Adach, W., Janikowski, K., Banach, M., Bielecka-Dabrowa, A. Menopause and women's cardiovascular health: is it really an obvious relationship? *Archives of Medical Science* **19**, 458–466 (2022). https://doi.org/10.5114/aoms/157308

Woods, N. F., Carr, M. C., Tao, E. Y., Taylor, H. J., Mitchell, E. S. Increased urinary cortisol levels during the menopausal transition. *Menopause* **13**, 212–221 (2006).

Chapter 2

Bailey, R. R. Goal setting and action planning for health behavior change. American Journal of Lifestyle Medicine 13, 615–618 (2017). https://doi.org/10.1177/1559827617729634

Gardner, S., Albee, D. *Study focuses on strategies for achieving goals, resolutions*. Press Releases 266 (2015). https://scholar.dominican.edu/news-releases/266

Razzaque, M. S. Magnesium: are we consuming enough? *Nutrients* **10**, 1863 (2018). https://doi.org/10.3390/nu10121863

Chapter 3

Australian Mushroom Growers Association. Vitamin D in mushrooms. *Australian Mushroom Growers Association* (n.d.). https://australianmushroomgrowers.com.au/health-benefits-of-mushrooms/vitamin-d-in-mushrooms/

Baker Heart & Diabetes Institute. Carbohydrates and glycaemic index (GI). *Baker Heart & Diabetes Institute* (n.d.). https://www.baker.edu.au/-/media/documents/fact-sheets/baker-institute-factsheet-carbohydrates-and-glycaemic-index.pdf

Berding, K., Vlckova, K., Marx, W., Schellekens, H., Stanton, C., Clarke, G., Jacka, F., Dinan, T. G., Cryan, J. F. Diet and the microbiota-gut-brain axis: sowing the seeds of good mental health. Advances in Nutrition 12, 1239–1285 (2021). https://doi.org/10.1093/advances/nmaa181

Better Health Channel. Menopause and osteoporosis. *Better Health Channel* (2024, August). https://www.betterhealth.vic.gov.au/health/conditionsandtreatments/menopause-and-osteoporosis

Cleveland Clinic. Ghrelin. *Cleveland Clinic* (2022, April). https://my.clevelandclinic.org/health/body/22804-ghrelin

Cleveland Clinic. Insulin resistance. *Cleveland Clinic* (2024, November). https://my.clevelandclinic.org/health/diseases/22206-insulin-resistance

Cleveland Clinic. Mediterranean diet. *Cleveland Clinic* (2024, July). https://my.clevelandclinic.org/health/articles/16037-mediterranean-diet

CSIRO. *Gut health and weight loss.* CSIRO (2019, January). [PDF]. Retrieved from: file:///Users/sgray6/Downloads/1800623%20Gut%20health%20and%20Weight%20loss%20Report%20%20Jan%202019FINALlrsinglepag%20(2).pdf

CSIRO. *Top nutrition tips for menopause.* CSIRO (2021, May). https://www.csiro.au/en/news/all/articles/2021/may/top-nutrition-tips-for-menopause

Decandia, D., Landolfo, E., Sacchetti, S., Gelfo, F., Petrosini, L., Cutuli, D. n-3 PUFA improve emotion and cognition during menopause: a systematic review. Nutrients 14, 1982 (2022). https://doi.org/10.3390/nu14091982

Erdélyi, A., Pálfi, E., Tűű, L., Nas, K., Szűcs, Z., Török, M., Jakab, A., Várbíró, S. The importance of nutrition in menopause and perimenopause – a review. *Nutrients* **16**, 27 (2023). https://doi.org/10.3390/nu16010027

Evans, M., Elliott, J. G., Sharma, P., Berman, R., Guthrie, N. The effect of synthetic genistein on menopause symptom management in healthy postmenopausal women: a multi-center, randomized, placebo-controlled study. *Maturitas* **68**, 189–196 (2011). https://www.maturitas.org/article/S0378-5122(10)00423-8/abstract

Fahey, J.W., Raphaely, M. (2025). The Impact of Sulforaphane on Sex-Specific Conditions and Hormone Balance: A Comprehensive Review. Applied Sciences, 15, 522. https://doi.org/10.3390/app15020522

Glazier, M. G., Bowman, M. A. A review of the evidence for the use of phytoestrogens as a replacement for traditional estrogen replacement therapy. *Archives of Internal Medicine* **161**, 1161–1172 (2001). https://jamanetwork.com/journals/jamainternalmedicine/fullarticle/648139

Guasch-Ferré, M., Willett. W. C. The Mediterranean diet and health: a comprehensive overview. Journal of Internal Medicine. 290, 3, 549-566 (2021). https://doi.org/10.1111/joim.13333

Hamad, M., Bajbouj, K., Taneera, J. The case for an estrogen–iron axis in health and disease. *Experimental and Clinical Endocrinology & Diabetes* **128**, 270–277 (2020). https://www.thieme-connect.de/products/ejournals/abstract/10.1055/a-0885-1677

REFERENCES

Harvard Health Publishing. *9 tips to boost your energy – naturally*. Harvard Medical School (2024, April). https://www.health.harvard.edu/healthbeat/9-tips-to-boost-your-energy-naturally

Health Direct Australia. *Vitamins and minerals explained*. Health Direct (2024, March). https://www.healthdirect.gov.au/vitamins-and-minerals-explained

Jacka, F. N., O'Neil, A., Opie, R., Itsiopoulos, C., Cotton, S., Mohebbi, M., Castle, D., Dash, S., Mihalopoulos, C., Chatterton, M. L., Brazionis, L., Dean, O. M., Hodge, A. M., Berk, M. A randomised controlled trial of dietary improvement for adults with major depression (the 'SMILES' trial). BMC Medicine **15**, 23 (2017). https://bmcmedicine.biomedcentral.com/articles/10.1186/s12916-017-0791-y

Jean Hailes for Women's Health. *Foods for menopause*. Jean Hailes (2024, December). https://www.jeanhailes.org.au/news/foods-for-menopause

Khaodhiar, L., Ricciotti, H. A., Li, L., Pan, W., Schickel, M., Zhou, J., Blackburn, G. L. Daidzein-rich isoflavone aglycones are potentially effective in reducing hot flashes in menopausal women. Menopause **15**, 125–132 (2008). https://pubmed.ncbi.nlm.nih.gov/18257146/

Kumar, S., Kaur, G. Intermittent fasting dietary restriction regimen negatively influences reproduction in young rats: a study of hypothalamo-hypophysial-gonadal axis. PLoS ONE **8**, e52416 (2013). https://doi.org/10.1371/journal.pone.0052416

Lee, S., Shu, X., Li, H., Yang, G., Cai, H., Wen, W., Ji, B., Gao, J., Gao, Y., Zheng, W. S. Adolescent and adult soy food intake and breast cancer risk: results from the Shanghai Women's Health Study. The American Journal of Clinical Nutrition 89, 6, 1920-6 (2009). https://doi.org/10.3945/ajcn.2008.27361

Lim, S., Moon, J. H., Shin, C. M., Jeong, D., Kim, B. Effect of *Lactobacillus sakei*, a probiotic derived from kimchi, on body fat in Koreans with obesity: a randomized controlled study. Endocrinology and Metabolism **35**, 425–434 (2020). https://doi.org/10.3803/EnM.2020.35.2.425

Maeng, Y. L., Beumer, A. Never fear, the gut bacteria are here: Estrogen and gut microbiome-brain axis interactions in fear extinction. International Journal of Psychophysiology **189**, 66–75 (2023). https://doi.org/10.1016/j.ijpsycho.2023.05.350

MedlinePlus. *Omega-3 fats – good for your heart*. MedlinePlus (2024, June). https://medlineplus.gov/ency/patientinstructions/000767.htm

McDonald D, Hyde E, Debelius JW, et al. American Gut: an Open Platform for Citizen Science Microbiome Research. mSystems 3, 10 (2018). https://journals.asm.org/doi/10.1128/msystems.00031-18

Młynarska, E., Hajdys, J., Czarnik, W., Fularski, P., Leszto, K., Majchrowicz, G., Lisińska, W., Rysz, J., Franczyk, B. The role of antioxidants in the therapy of cardiovascular diseases – A literature review. *Nutrients* **16**, 2587 (2024). https://www.eurekaselect.com/article/69293

Nagata, C., Takatsuka, N., Kawakami, N., Shimizu, H. Soy product intake and hot flashes in Japanese women: Results from a community-based prospective study. *American Journal of Epidemiology* **153**, 790–793 (2001). https://academic.oup.com/aje/article-abstract/153/8/790/106842?redirectedFrom=fulltext

National Cancer Institute. *Cruciferous vegetables and cancer prevention.* National Cancer Institute (2012, June). https://www.cancer.gov/about-cancer/causes-prevention/risk/diet/cruciferous-vegetables-fact-sheet

National Health and Medical Research Council. *Fat, Salt, Sugars and Alcohol. Eat for Health* (n.d.). https://www.eatforhealth.gov.au/food-essentials/fat-salt-sugars-and-alcohol

Olive Wellness Institute. Health benefits of extra virgin olive oil. (2025, April). https://olivewellnessinstitute.org/extra-virgin-olive-oil/health-benefits-of-extra-virgin-olive-oil/

Schulman, I. H., Aranda, P., Raij, L., Veronesi, M., Aranda, F. J., Martin, R. Surgical menopause increases salt sensitivity of blood pressure. *Hypertension* **47**, 1168–1174 (2006). https://doi.org/10.1161/01.HYP.0000218857.67880.7

Simpson, S. J., Raubenheimer, D., Black, K. I., Conigrave, A. D. Weight gain during the menopause transition: evidence for a mechanism dependent on protein leverage. BJOG **130**, 4–10 (2023). https://doi.org/10.1111/1471-0528.17290

Sleep Foundation. *Alcohol and Sleep.* Sleep Foundation (2024, May). https://www.sleepfoundation.org/nutrition/alcohol-and-sleep#:~:text=pauses%20in%20breathing.-,Insomnia,insomnia%20symptoms%20when%20they%20drink

Song, D. K., Kim, Y. W. Beneficial effects of intermittent fasting: a narrative review. *Journal of Yeungnam Medical Science* **40**, 4–11 (2023). https://doi.org/10.12701/jyms.2022.00010

Wiciński, M., Gębalski, J., Gołębiewski, J., Malinowski, B. Probiotics for the treatment of overweight and obesity in humans – A review of clinical trials. *Microorganisms* **8**, 1148 (2020). https://doi.org/10.3390/microorganisms8081148

Yang, W., Cui, K., Li, X., Zhao, J., Zeng, Z., Song, R., Qi, X., Xu, W. Effect of polyphenols on cognitive function: evidence from population-based studies and clinical trials. *The Journal of Nutrition Health and Aging* **25**, 1190–1204 (2021). https://doi.org/10.1007/s12603-021-1685-4

Chapter 4

Apgar, B. S., Greenberg, G. Using progestins in clinical practice. American Family Physician 62, 1839–1850 (2000). https://pubmed.ncbi.nlm.nih.gov/11057840/

REFERENCES

Asi, N., Mohammed, K., Haydour, Q., Gionfriddo, M. R., Vargas, O. L., Prokop, L. J., Faubion, S. S., Murad, M. H. Progesterone vs. synthetic progestins and the risk of breast cancer: a systematic review and meta-analysis. Systematic Reviews 5, 121 (2016). https://systematicreviewsjournal.biomedcentral.com/articles/10.1186/s13643-016-0294-5

Better Health Channel. Strong relationships, strong health. *Better Health Channel* (n.d.). https://www.betterhealth.vic.gov.au/health/healthyliving/Strong-relationships-strong-health

Better Health Channel. Strong relationships, strong health. *Better Health Channel* (n.d.). https://www.betterhealth.vic.gov.au/health/healthyliving/Strong-relationships-strong-health

Breastcancer.org. Using HRT (Hormone Replacement Therapy). *Breastcancer.org* (2024, January). https://www.breastcancer.org/risk/risk-factors/using-hormone-replacement-therapy

Canadian Cancer Society. All about hormone replacement therapy (HRT). *Canadian Cancer Society* (n.d.). https://cancer.ca/en/cancer-information/reduce-your-risk/understand-hormones/all-about-hormone-replacement-therapy-hrt

Carmody, J. F., Crawford, S., Salmoirago-Blotcher, E., Leung, K., Churchill, L., Olendzki, N. Mindfulness training for coping with hot flashes: results of a randomized trial. Menopause 18, 611–620 (2011). https://journals.lww.com/menopausejournal/abstract/2011/06000/mindfulness_training_for_coping_with_hot_flashes_.6.aspx

Duygu, A., Ulusu, N. N. The possible role of the endocrine disrupting chemicals on the premature and early menopause associated with the altered oxidative stress metabolism. Frontiers in Endocrinology 14 (2023). https://doi.org/10.3389/fendo.2023.1081704

Figueiro, M. G., Steverson, B., Heerwagen, J., Kampschroer, K., Hunter, C. M., Gonzales, K., Plitnick, B., Rea, M. S. The impact of daytime light exposures on sleep and mood in office workers. *Sleep Health* **3**, 204–215 (2017). https://www.sleephealthjournal.org/article/S2352-7218(17)30041-4/abstract

Gordon, J. L., Girdler, S. S., Meltzer-Brody, S. E., Stika, C. S., Thurston, R. C., Clark, C. T., Prairie, B. A., Moses-Kolko, E., Joffe, H., Wisner, K. L. Ovarian hormone fluctuation, neurosteroids, and HPA axis dysregulation in perimenopausal depression: a novel heuristic model. *American Journal of Psychiatry* **172**, 227–236 (2015). https://doi.org/10.1176/appi.ajp.2014.14070918

Endocrine Society. *Plastics, EDCs & health: Authoritative guide.* Endocrine Society (2020,

Endocrine Society. *What you can do about EDCs.* Endocrine Society (n.d.). https://www.endocrine.org/topics/edc/what-you-can-do#

Health Direct Australia. *Hormone replacement therapy* (HRT). Health Direct (2024, February). https://www.healthdirect.gov.au/hormone-replacement-therapy

Hurtado, M. D., Tama, E., Fansa, S., Ghusn, W., Anazco, D., Acosta, A., Faubion, S. S., Shufelt, C. L. Weight loss response to semaglutide in postmenopausal women with and without hormone therapy use. *Menopause* **31**, 266–274 (2024). https://journals.lww.com/menopausejournal/fulltext/2024/04000/weight_loss_response_to_semaglutide_in.4.aspx

Jean Hailes for Women's Health. *Treatments for menopause*. Jean Hailes (2025, April). https://www.jeanhailes.org.au/health-a-z/menopause/menopause-management#non-hormone-treatments-for-menopause

Lederman, S., Ottery, F. D., Cano, A., Santoro, N., Shapiro, M., Stute, P., Thurston, R. C., English, M., Franklin, C., Lee, M., Neal-Perry, G. Fezolinetant for treatment of moderate-to-severe vasomotor symptoms associated with menopause (SKYLIGHT 1): a phase 3 randomised controlled study. *Lancet* **401**, 1091–1102 (2023). https://www.thelancet.com/journals/lancet/article/PIIS0140-6736(23)00085-5/abstract

Magraith, K., Jang, C. Management of menopause. *Australian Prescriber* **46**, 48–53 (2023). https://australianprescriber.tg.org.au/articles/management-of-menopause.html

Magraith, K., Stuckey, B. Making choices at menopause. *Australian Journal of General Practice* **48**, (2019). https://www1.racgp.org.au/ajgp/2019/july/making-choices-at-menopause

NHS. *Benefits and Risks of Hormone Replacement Therapy* (HRT). NHS (2023, February). https://www.nhs.uk/medicines/hormone-replacement-therapy-hrt/benefits-and-risks-of-hormone-replacement-therapy-hrt/#:~:text=If%20you%27ve%20had%20breast,after%20you%20stop%20taking%20it

Reddy, V., McCarthy, M., Raval, A. P. Xenoestrogens impact brain estrogen receptor signaling during the female lifespan: a precursor to neurological disease? *Neurobiology of Disease* **163**, 105596 (2021). https://doi.org/10.1016/j.nbd.2021.105596

Shaw, J. M., Snow, C. M. Weighted vest exercise improves indices of fall risk in older women. *The Journals of Gerontology Series A: Biological Sciences and Medical Sciences* **53**, M53–M58 (1998). https://doi.org/10.1093/gerona/53A.1.M53

Snow, C. M., Shaw, J. M., Winters, K. M., Witzke, K. A. Long-term exercise using weighted vests prevents hip bone loss in postmenopausal women. *The Journals of Gerontology Series A: Biological Sciences and Medical Sciences* **55**, M489–M491 (2000). https://doi.org/10.1093/gerona/55.9.M489

Sood, R., Kuhle, C. L., Kapoor, E., Thielen, J. M., Frohmader, K. S., Mara, K. C., Faubion, S. S. Association of mindfulness and stress with menopausal symptoms

REFERENCES

in midlife women. *Climacteric* **22**, 377–382 (2019). https://doi.org/10.1080/1369 7137.2018.1551344

Srisaphonphusitti, L., Manimmanakorn, N., Manimmanakorn, A., Hamlin, M. J. Effects of whole body vibration exercise combined with weighted vest in older adults: a randomized controlled trial. BMC *Geriatrics* **22**, 911 (2022). https://bmcgeriatr.biomedcentral.com/articles/10.1186/s12877-022-03593-4

Sung, M. K., Lee, U. S., Ha, N. H., Koh, E., Yang, H. J. A potential association of meditation with menopausal symptoms and blood chemistry in healthy women: a pilot cross-sectional study. *Medicine (Baltimore)* **99**, e22048 (2020). https://journals.lww.com/md-journal/fulltext/2020/09040/a_potential_association_of_meditation_with.77.aspx

Turakitwanakan, W., Mekseepralard, C., Busarakumtragul, P. Effects of mindfulness meditation on serum cortisol of medical students. *The Journal of the Medical Association of Thailand* **96** (Suppl 1), S90–S95 (2013). https://pubmed.ncbi.nlm.nih.gov/23724462/

Vogel, L. Early hormone replacement therapy may yield benefits, researchers say. *Canadian Medical Association Journal* **183**, E1237–E1238 (2011). https://doi.org/10.1503/cmaj.109-4041

Chapter 5

Álvarez-Arraño, V. Martín-Peláez, S. Effects of probiotics and synbiotics on weight loss in subjects with overweight or obesity: a systematic review. Nutrients 13, 3627 (2021). https://doi.org/10.3390/nu13103627

Antonio, J., et al. Common questions and misconceptions about creatine supplementation: what does the scientific evidence really show? Journal of the International Society of Sports Nutrition 18, 13 (2021). https://doi.org/10.1186/s12970-021-00412-w

Andrews, R., et al. Evaluating the effects of probiotics on menopause-specific health outcomes: a systematic review & meta-analysis. OSF Preprints (2023). https://doi.org/10.31219/osf.io/a7hky

Australian Menopause Society. Complementary and herbal medicines for hot flushes. *Australian Menopause Society* (2018, January). https://www.menopause.org.au/images/stories/infosheets/docs/AMS_Complementary_and_Herbal_Therapies_Hot_Flushes.pdf

Black Dog Institute. St John's wort as a depression treatment. *Black Dog Institute* (n.d.). https://www.blackdoginstitute.org.au/wp-content/uploads/2022/06/St-Johns-Worts-treatment.pdf

British Menopause Society. Non-hormonal based treatments for menopausal symptoms. *British Menopause Society* (2024, September). https://thebms.org.

uk/wp-content/uploads/2024/09/04-BMS-ConsensusStatement-Non-hormonal-based-treatments-SEPT2024-A.pdf

Cancelo-Hidalgo, M. J., Castelo-Branco, C., Palacios, S., Haya-Palazuelos, J., Ciria-Recasens, M., Manasanch, J., Pérez-Edo, L. Tolerability of different oral iron supplements: a systematic review. Current Medical Research and Opinion 29, 291–303 (2013). https://doi.org/10.1185/03007995.2012.761599

Chang, J. L., Montalto, M. B., Heger, P. W., Thiemann, E., Rettenberger, R., Wacker, J. Rheum rhaponticum extract (ERr 731): postmarketing data on safety surveillance and consumer complaints. Integrative Medicine (Encinitas, Calif.) 15, 34–39 (2016). https://pmc.ncbi.nlm.nih.gov/articles/PMC4982646/

Chen, Q., Wang, H., Wang, G., Zhao, J., Chen, H., Lu, X., Chen, W. Lactic acid bacteria: a promising tool for menopausal health management in women. Nutrients 14, 4466 (2022). https://doi.org/10.3390/nu14214466

Chopin, L. B. Vitex agnus castus essential oil and menopausal balance: a research update. Complementary Therapies in Nursing and Midwifery 9, 157–160 (2003). https://doi.org/10.1016/S1353-6117(03)00020-9

Cleveland Clinic. Black cohosh oral dosage forms. *Cleveland Clinic* (n.d.). https://my.clevelandclinic.org/health/drugs/18489-black-cohosh-oral-dosage-forms

Cleveland Clinic. Vitamin B complex tablets or capsules. *Cleveland Clinic* (n.d.). https://my.clevelandclinic.org/health/drugs/23803-vitamin-b-complex-tablets-or-capsules

Cordingley, D. M., Cornish, S. M. Omega-3 fatty acids for the management of osteoarthritis: a narrative review. Nutrients 14, 3362 (2022). https://doi.org/10.3390/nu14163362

Daniele, C., Thompson Coon, J., Pittler, M. H., Ernst, E. Vitex agnus castus: a systematic review of adverse events. Drug Safety 28, 319–332 (2005). https://link.springer.com/article/10.2165/00002018-200528040-00004

Decandia, D., Landolfo, E., Sacchetti, S., Gelfo, F., Petrosini, L., Cutuli, D. n-3 PUFA improve emotion and cognition during menopause: a systematic review. Nutrients 14, 1982 (2022). https://doi.org/10.3390/nu14091982

Eatemadnia, A., Ansari, S., Abedi, P., Najar, S. The effect of Hypericum perforatum on postmenopausal symptoms and depression: a randomized controlled trial. Complementary Therapies in Medicine 45, 109–113 (2019). https://doi.org/10.1016/j.ctim.2019.05.028

Fröhlich, E., Wahl, R. Thyroid autoimmunity: role of anti-thyroid antibodies in thyroid and extra-thyroidal diseases. *Frontiers in Immunology* **9**, 521 (2017). https://www.frontiersin.org/journals/immunology/articles/10.3389/fimmu.2017.00521/full

Gopal, S., Ajgaonkar, A., Kanchi, P., Kaundinya, A., Thakare, V., Chauhan, S., Langade, D. Effect of an ashwagandha (*Withania somnifera*) root extract on climacteric

REFERENCES

symptoms in women during perimenopause: a randomized, double-blind, placebo-controlled study. *Journal of Obstetrics and Gynaecology Research* **47**, 4414–4425 (2021). https://doi.org/10.1111/jog.15030

Hasper, I., Ventskovskiy, B. M., Rettenberger, R., Heger, P. W., Riley, D. S., Kaszkin-Bettag, M. Long-term efficacy and safety of the special extract ERr 731 of *Rheum rhaponticum* in perimenopausal women with menopausal symptoms. *Menopause* **16**, 117–131 (2009). https://journals.lww.com/menopausejournal/abstract/2009/16010/long_term_efficacy_and_safety_of_the_special.21.aspx

Health Direct Australia. *Magnesium*. Health Direct (2023, May). https://www.healthdirect.gov.au/magnesium

Health Direct Australia. *Melatonin*. Health Direct (2023, July). https://www.healthdirect.gov.au/melatonin

Hedaoo, K., Badge, A. K., Tiwade, Y. R., Bankar, N. J., Mishra, V. H. Exploring the efficacy and safety of black cohosh (*Cimicifuga racemosa*) in menopausal symptom management. *Journal of Mid-life Health* **15**, 5–11 (2024). https://journals.lww.com/jomh/fulltext/2024/15010/exploring_the_efficacy_and_safety_of_black_cohosh.3.aspx

Juneja, K., Bhuchakra, H. P., Sadhukhan, S., Mehta, I., Niharika, A., Thareja, S., Nimmakayala, T., Sahu, S. Creatine supplementation in depression: a review of mechanisms, efficacy, clinical outcomes, and future directions. *Cureus* **16**, e71638 (2024). https://www.cureus.com/articles/301707-creatine-supplementation-in-depression-a-review-of-mechanisms-efficacy-clinical-outcomes-and-future-directions#!/

Kanadys, W., Barańska, A., Błaszczuk, A., Polz-Dacewicz, M., Drop, B., Kanecki, K., Malm, M. Evaluation of clinical meaningfulness of red clover (*Trifolium pratense* L.) extract to relieve hot flushes and menopausal symptoms in peri- and post-menopausal women: a systematic review and meta-analysis of randomized controlled trials. *Nutrients* **13**, 1258 (2021). https://doi.org/10.3390/nu13041258

Kazemi, F., Masoumi, S. Z., Shayan, A., Oshvandi, K. The effect of evening primrose oil capsule on hot flashes and night sweats in postmenopausal women: a single-blind randomized controlled trial. *Journal of Menopausal Medicine* **27**, 8–14 (2021). https://e-jmm.org/DOIx.php?id=10.6118/jmm.20033

Komesaroff, P. A., Black, C. V., Cable, V., Sudhir, K. Effects of wild yam extract on menopausal symptoms, lipids and sex hormones in healthy menopausal women. *Climacteric* **4**, 144–150 (2001). https://pubmed.ncbi.nlm.nih.gov/11428178/

Liu, L., Luo, P., Wen, P., Xu, P. The role of magnesium in the pathogenesis of osteoporosis. *Frontiers in Endocrinology* **15**, 1406248 (2024). https://doi.org/10.3389/fendo.2024.1406248

Liu, Y. R., Jiang, Y. L., Huang, R. Q., Yang, J. Y., Xiao, B. K., Dong, J. X. *Hypericum perforatum* L. preparations for menopause: A meta-analysis of efficacy and safety. *Climacteric* **17**, 325–335 (2014). https://doi.org/10.3109/13697137.2013.861814

Mayo Clinic. *Can ashwagandha supplements really provide stress relief?* Mayo Clinic (2023, June). https://mcpress.mayoclinic.org/mental-health/ashwagandha-supplements/

Mohammady, M., Janani, L., Jahanfar, S., Mousavi, M. S. Effect of omega-3 supplements on vasomotor symptoms in menopausal women: A systematic review and meta-analysis. *European Journal of Obstetrics & Gynecology and Reproductive Biology* **228**, 295–302 (2018). https://www.ejog.org/article/S0301-2115(18)30335-X/abstract

National Center for Complementary and Integrative Health. *Ashwagandha*. NCCIH (2023, March). https://www.nccih.nih.gov/health/ashwagandha#:~:text=In%20some%20individuals%2C%20ashwagandha%20preparations,not%20be%20used%20while%20breastfeeding

National Center for Complementary and Integrative Health. *St. John's Wort*. NCCIH (2025, May). https://www.nccih.nih.gov/health/st-johns-wort

National Institutes for Health. Office of Dietary Supplements. *Ashwagandha: Is it Helpful for Stress, Anxiety or Sleep?* NIH ODS (2025, May). https://ods.od.nih.gov/factsheets/Ashwagandha-HealthProfessional/#:~:text=Several%20randomized%2C%20placebo%2Dcontrolled%20clinical,8%2C20%2C45%5D

National Library of Medicine. *Magnesium*. NLM (2023, February). https://www.ncbi.nlm.nih.gov/books/NBK519036/#:~:text=For%20contraindications%2C%20factors%20to%20consider,which%20can%20lead%20to%20toxicity

O'Keefe, E. L., O'Keefe, J. H., Abuissa, H., Metzinger, M., Murray, E., Franco, G., Lavie, C. J., Harris, W. S. Omega-3 and risk of atrial fibrillation: vagally-mediated double-edged sword. *Progress in Cardiovascular Diseases* **30**, S0033-0620(24)00168-3 (2024). https://doi.org/10.1016/j.pcad.2024.11.003

Pasupathy, E., Kandasamy, R., Thomas, K., Basheer, A. Alternate day versus daily oral iron for treatment of iron deficiency anemia: a randomized controlled trial. *Scientific Reports* **13**, 1818 (2023). https://www.nature.com/articles/s41598-023-29034-9

Porri, D., Biesalski, H. K., Limitone, A., Bertuzzo, L., Cena, H. Effect of magnesium supplementation on women's health and well-being. *NFS Journal* **23**, 30–36 (2021). https://doi.org/10.1016/j.nfs.2021.03.003

Rawji, A., Peltier, M. R., Mourtzanakis, K., Awan, S., Rana, J., Pothen, N. J., Afzal, S. Examining the effects of supplemental magnesium on self-reported anxiety and sleep quality: a systematic review. *Cureus* **16**(4), e59317 (2024). https://

REFERENCES

www.cureus.com/articles/237565-examining-the-effects-of-supplemental-magnesium-on-self-reported-anxiety-and-sleep-quality-a-systematic-review#!/

Sanders, M. E., Merenstein, D. J., Ouwehand, A. C., Reid, G., Salminen, S., Cabana, M. D., Paraskevakos, G., Leyer, G. Probiotic use in at-risk populations. *Journal of the American Pharmacists Association* **56**, 680–686 (2016). https://www.japha.org/article/S1544-3191(16)30732-4/fulltext

Stoffel, N. U., Zeder, C., Brittenham, G. M., Moretti, D., Zimmermann, M. B. Iron absorption from supplements is greater with alternate day than with consecutive day dosing in iron-deficient anemic women. *Haematologica* **105**, 1232–1239 (2020). https://doi.org/10.3324/haematol.2019.220830

Taku, K., Melby, M. K., Nishi, N., Omori, T., Kurzer, M. S. Soy isoflavones for osteoporosis: an evidence-based approach. *Maturitas* **70**, 333–338 (2011). https://www.maturitas.org/article/S0378-5122(11)00320-3/abstract

Tardy, A. L., Pouteau, E., Marquez, D., Yilmaz, C., Scholey, A. Vitamins and minerals for energy, fatigue and cognition: a narrative review of the biochemical and clinical evidence. *Nutrients* **12**, 228 (2020). https://doi.org/10.3390/nu12010228

Uebelhack, R., Blohmer, J. U., Graubaum, H. J., Busch, R., Gruenwald, J., Wernecke, K. D. Black cohosh and St. John's wort for climacteric complaints: a randomized trial. *Obstetrics & Gynecology* **107**, 247–255 (2006). https://journals.lww.com/greenjournal/abstract/2006/02000/black_cohosh_and_st__john_s_wort_for_climacteric.8.aspx

Wang, J., Gaman, M. A., Albadawi, N. I., Salem, A., Kord-Varkaneh, H., Okunade, K. S., Alomar, O., Al-Badawi, I. A., Abu-Zaid, A. Does omega-3 fatty acid supplementation have favorable effects on the lipid profile in postmenopausal women? A systematic review and dose-response meta-analysis of randomized controlled trials. *Clinical Therapeutics* **45**, e74–e87 (2023). https://www.clinicaltherapeutics.com/article/S0149-2918(22)00415-5/pdf

Yamadera, W., Inagawa, K., Chiba, S., Bannai, M., Takahashi, M., Nakayama, K. Glycine ingestion improves subjective sleep quality in human volunteers, correlating with polysomnographic changes. *Sleep and Biological Rhythms* **25**, 126–131 (2007). https://doi.org/10.1111/j.1479-8425.2007.00262.x

Yaralizadeh, M., Nezamivand-Chegini, S., Shahnaz, N., Forough, N., Parvin, A. Effectiveness of magnesium on menstrual symptoms among dysmenorrheal college students: a randomized controlled trial. *International Journal of Women's Health and Reproduction Sciences* **12**, 70–76 (2020). https://www.ijwhr.net/pdf/pdf_IJWHR_624.pdf

Zhang, C., Hu, Q., Li, S., Dai, F., Qian, W., Hewlings, S., Yan, T., Wang, Y. A Magtein®, magnesium L-threonate-based formula improves brain cognitive functions in healthy Chinese adults. *Nutrients* **14**, 5235 (2022). https://doi.org/10.3390/nu14245235

Zhang, L., Shang, F., Liu, C., Zhai, X. The correlation between iodine and metabolism: a review. *Frontiers in Nutrition* **11**, 1346452 (2024). https://doi.org/10.3389/fnut.2024.1346452

Bonus Chapter

Liu, J., Feng, W., Peng, C. A song of ice and fire: Cold and hot properties of traditional Chinese medicines. *Frontiers in Pharmacology* **11**, 598744 (2021). https://doi.org/10.3389/fphar.2020.598744

ABOUT THE AUTHOR

SARAH GRAY is one of Australia's leading dual-qualified health professionals in pharmacy and nutrition, holding a Bachelor of Pharmacy (with Honours) from Monash University and a Master of Human Nutrition from Deakin University. She is a registered pharmacist with the Australian Health Practitioner Regulation Agency (AHPRA), a registered nutritionist with the Nutrition Society of Australia, and a MyMT™ Certified Menopause Lifestyle Practitioner.

With over 25 years of experience in the health and wellness industry, her holistic approach focuses on supplements and science-based solutions for perimenopause and menopause. Sarah has developed a proven framework for implementing science-based solutions to manage the symptoms of perimenopause. Her philosophy is based on the multifactorial nature of health – being made up of the foods you eat, medicines or supplements you take, and how you move and look after your body and mind. A trusted thought leader, Sarah has appeared on Channel 10's *My Market Kitchen* and is a recognised voice across radio, print, digital media and podcasts. She is also a regular contributor to leading podcasts, health blogs and publications.

@the_nutrition_pharmacist

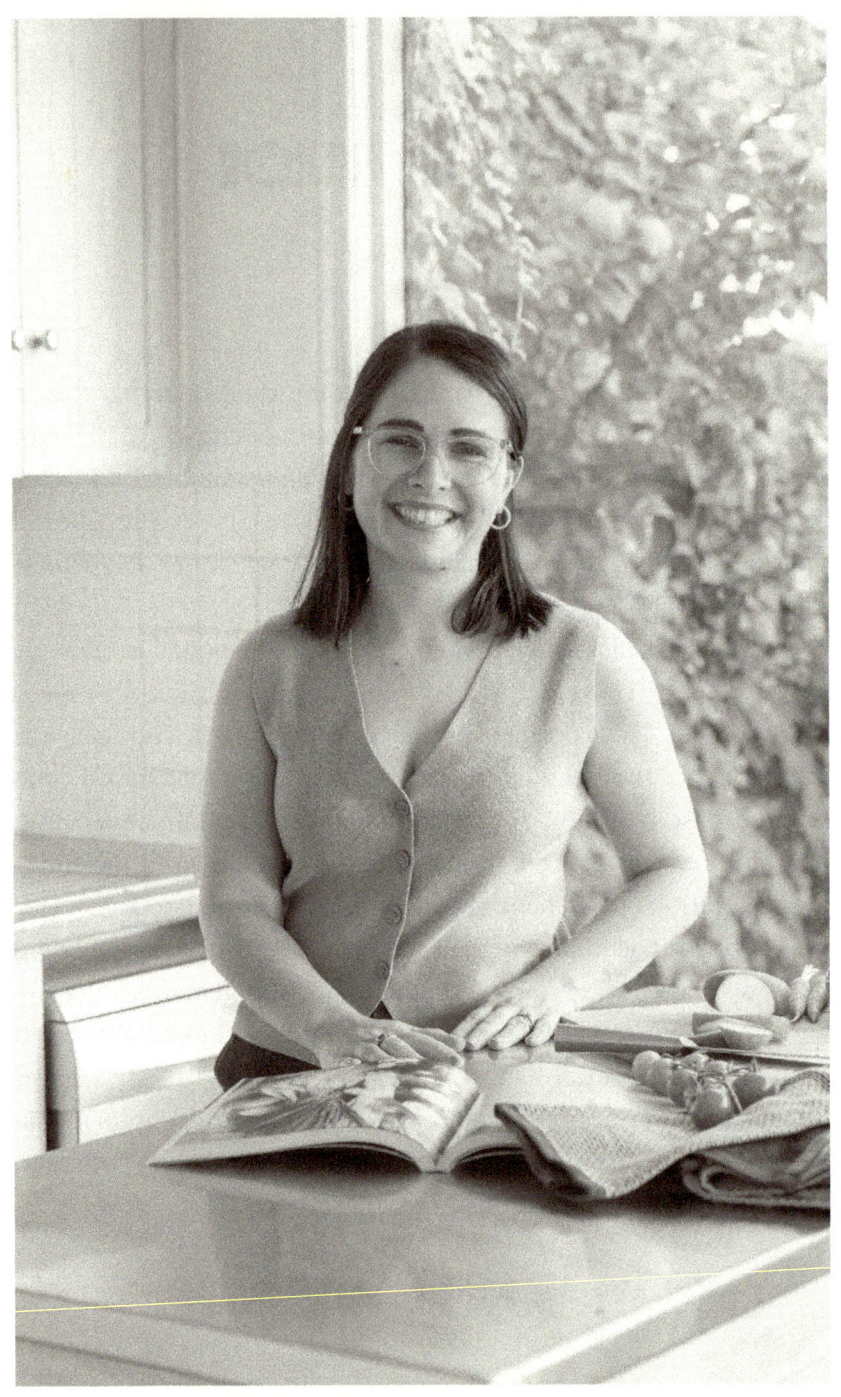

www.ingramcontent.com/pod-product-compliance
Lightning Source LLC
Chambersburg PA
CBHW031148020426
42333CB00013B/563